Zithromax-N
in chest

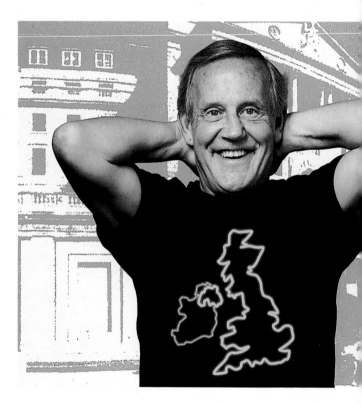

tionally trusted
nfections

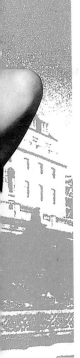

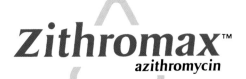
azithromycin

Simply effective in chest infections

Full prescribing information is available on
request from Richborough Pharmaceuticals.
A Division of Pfizer Ltd, Sandwich, Kent CT13 9NJ.
Legal category: POM.

RICHBOROUGH™
PHARMACEUTICALS
A Division of Pfizer Ltd., Sandwich, Kent CT13 9NJ

70730 September 1995

Copyright © 1995 Times Mirror International Publishers Limited

Published in 1995 by Mosby-Wolfe, an imprint of Times Mirror International Publishers Limited

Printed in Spain by Grafos S.A. arte sobre papel, Barcelona, Spain

ISBN 0 7234 1997 3 (hardback edition)

ISBN 0 7234 2127-7 (paperback edition)

For full details of all Times Mirror International Publishers Limited titles, please write to Times Mirror International Publishers Limited, Lynton House, 7–12 Tavistock Square, London WC1H 9LB, England.

A CIP catalogue record for this book is available from the British Library.

Library of Congress Cataloging-in-Publication Data has been applied for.

ACKNOWLEDGEMENTS

It would have been impossible to illustrate so many aspects of infection without the generosity and support of numerous friends and colleagues, who have provided photographs from their collections. We are most grateful to them for the following illustrations:

Dr June Almeida, **374**; Dr J. Bell, **144**; Professor C.P. Beattie, Professor J.K.A. Beverley and the Department of Photography, the United Sheffield Hospitals, **471–73, 475, 477–8**; Dr Isobel Beswick, **31**; the late Dr A. Bloom, **33** and **51**; Dr Jean Bradley, **1, 2, 37–9, 60, 112, 125, 481**; the late Dr R.T. Brain, **302**; the late Dr E.H. Brown, **118, 126, 268, 367**; Dr G. Laing Brown, **231–2**; Dr A.D.M. Bryceson, **156, 159**; Dr D.C. MacDonald Burns, **209**; Dr S. Burns, **329, 342**; Dr K.C. Carstairs and the Editor of the *Proceedings of the Royal Society of Medicine*, **237–8**; Dr L.S. Carstairs, **233–6**; Mr G.S.J. Chessell, Dr M.J. Jamieson, Mr R.A. Morton, Dr J.C. Petrie and Dr H.M.A. Towler, **150**; the late Dr A.B. Christie, **239, 444**; Mr M. Croughan, **135–7, 350**; Mr C. Daniels, **448**; Professor S. Darougar, **190–1**; Dr B. Dhillon, **344, 347–8**; Mr D. Downton, **127**; the late Professor J.A. Dudgeon and the Hospital for Sick Children, London, who retain the copyright, **398–9, 409, 411, 414**; Dr A.J. Duggan, **179**; Professor K.R. Dumbell, **277–8**; Dr G.J. Ebrahim, **466**; Dr Anne M. Field and Mr A. Porter, **213, 320, 359, 416, 441**; Dr W.J.D. Fleming, **308**; Dr T.H. Flewett, **101**; Dr J.A. Forbes, **166**; Ms Sue Ford, Western Eye Hospital, **142**; Dr G.A. Gresham, **169, 482, 511**; Mr M.D.F. Grindley, **84**; Dr S. Haider, **293**; Dr M. Hendry, **83**; Professors H.M. Gilles, A.J.Radford and W. Peters, **151**; the late Dr K.K. Hussain, **98**; Dr W.M. Jamieson, **12, 80, 119, 121, 171, 381, 442–3, 445, 447**; Mr J.J. Kanski, **187**; Dr T. Kawasaki, **501–6, 508–9**; Dr S.G. Lamb, **7, 26, 218, 295, 393, 476, 494**; Professor H.P. Lambert, **415, 479–80**; Dr J.H. Lawson, **177**; Dr J.J. Linehan, **382, 390, 406**; Dr S. Lucas, **153–4, 460, 469–70**; Dr J. Luder, **66, 394**; Mrs S.D. Marston, **307**; Dr J.M. Medlock, **9–11, 34, 44, 114, 164**; Mr I. McCaul, **51**; Dr A.B. Maclaren, **139**; Dr G.D.W. McKendrick, **53, 71, 165, 205**; Dr W.F.T. McMath, the late Dr K.K. Hussain and the Editor and Publisher of the *British Medical Journal*, **357–8**; Dr E. Montuschi, **77**; Dr J.McC. Murdoch and Dr J.A. Gray, **21, 45**; Dr R.O. Murray, **96–7, 99**; Professor I.C.S. Norman, **408**; Dr R.J. Olds, **40, 78, 109, 111, 113, 129, 163, 174**; the late Dr E.P. O'Sullivan, **47–8, 79, 81, 223, 397, 412, 431**; Dr G. Pampiglione, **396**; Dr J.D.J. Parker, **299–300**; Dr G.H. Prentice, **306**; Dr J.I. Pugh, **281–2, 286, 340**; Dr C.S. Ratnatunga, **194, 208**; Dr G.H. Ree, **210–11**; Dr D. Taylor-Robinson, **214–15**; Dr G. Sangster and Dr J.A. Gray, **86–7**; Dr C. Santosh, **345–6, 352–3**; Professor P. Scheuer, **454**; Professor C. Scully, **435**; Mr J.C. Snale, **436**; Dr O.D. Standen, **178**; Dr J.H. Stern, **303–4, 343**; Dr J. Stevenson, **420–2**; the late Dr R.N.P. Sutton, **188, 279–80, 360, 362, 364, 375–6, 417–18, 438**; Dr Frances Tatnell, **355**; Dr M.M. Esiri and Dr A.H. Tomlinson, and the Editor of the

Journal of The Neurological Sciences, **244**; Dr A.H. Tomlinson, **284–5**; Dr J.M. Vetters and the Department of Pathology, University of Glasgow, **32**, **43**, **92–3**, **122–3**, **175**, **216–17**, **243**, **245**, **283**, **305**, **321–2**, **341**, **361**, **377–80**, **474**; Dr R.V. Walley, **176**; the late Dr J.F. Warin, **105–6**; Professor D.A. Warrell, **167**, **437**, **439–40**; Dr D.I. Weiss and the Editor of *American Journal of Diseases of Childhood*, **413**; Department of Pathology, Whittington Hospital, London, **62**; Dr A. Wightman, **148–9**, **337**; Dr P.H.A. Willcox, **512–13**; Dr I. Zamiri, **115**, **117**.

We wish to express special thanks to our colleagues, the late Dr A.M. Ramsay and Dr Hillas Smith, in The Infectious Diseases Department of The Royal Free Hospital, and to Dr J.I. Pugh of the City Hospital, St Albans for their help and advice in preparing this atlas. We are also indebted to many other colleagues at The Royal Free Hospital and to Mr Martin Jones of the Photographic Department of the North London Group of Hospitals. Many of the colour reproductions were obtained from members of the former Association for the Study of Infectious Disease, to whom we are most grateful. Every endeavour has been made to identify the source of the illustrations, but if any mistake has been made we offer our sincere apologies.

CONTENTS

PREFACE

The twentieth century has witnessed tremendous advances in the understanding of infectious disease, but many problems remain. With the natural ebb and flow of infection some old plagues have vanished, while others have been routed by rising standards of living and great advances in preventive medicine. Yet experience teaches that there is no final victory over infection, for elimination of one problem highlights another, and the delicate balance between man and microorganism remains. Moreover, the speed of air travel is such that banished infections can readily invade from distant lands. Constant vigilance is essential, but few undergraduates have the opportunity to study infectious disease at the bedside and most enter their profession ill-equipped to recognise even common infections, which form such an important part of everyday practice.

This atlas endeavours to provide the student and newly qualified doctor with a guide to the diagnosis of the common exanthemata, and the experienced physician with clinical photographs of less common though important diseases. It is not feasible to encompass the whole of the subject in one atlas, for many conditions are rare and others do not lend themselves to photographic illustration. Emphasis has been placed on the clinical aspects of disease, but this would be incomplete without a brief account of the causative organism and the relevant pathology. The texts accompanying the illustrations are of necessity short but, when read in sequence, are intended to give a simple, coherent account of each disease. When size is important in an illustration the relevant information is provided in the text.

Since the first edition was published in 1974 there have been many changes in the pattern of infectious disease. Smallpox has been banished from the world, new diseases such as AIDS have emerged, while old enemies such as tuberculosis have re-established a hold in many countries. Basic knowledge has expanded greatly and diagnostic investigations have become increasingly sophisticated. In this third edition we have revised the text and have introduced new sections on tuberculosis and AIDS. Many new illustrations have been included and old ones replaced, but the format of the atlas is unchanged.

BACTERIAL AND FUNGAL INFECTIONS
Streptococcal infection

The genus *Streptococcus* consists of Gram-positive, chain-forming cocci; most are aerobic, a few anaerobic. Beta, alpha and non-haemolytic groups are recognised but the main differentiation of streptococci, especially applicable to beta-haemolytic strains, is by the character of the cell-wall polysaccharide antigen (Lancefield grouping). Those beta-haemolytic streptococci belonging to Lancefield group A are also known as *Streptococcus pyogenes*. Most human infections are caused by this organism, which is associated with such varied diseases as tonsillitis, scarlet fever, erysipelas and impetigo. Sensitisation to the organism gives rise to erythema nodosum, acute rheumatic fever, or to acute glomerulonephritis. Other superficial protein antigens (M, T and R) are also present in *Strep. pyogenes* and are useful for epidemiological studies. M antigens are important virulence factors and induce type-specific immunity; certain types are recognised as nephritogenic. Several exotoxins may be produced by *Strep. pyogenes*.

- Streptolysin O: damages cells by binding to cholesterol in membranes; cardiotoxic for many animals, possibly including humans; potent antigen.

- Streptolysin S: also a haemolysin but its mode of action is not understood; toxic to leucocytes; not antigenic.

- Deoxyribonuclease (streptodornase), streptokinase, hyaluronidase; all probably contribute to spread of infection through tissues.

- Erythrogenic toxins: produced by some strains; three serotypes, A, B, and C; antigenic.

Viridans streptococci are a major cause of bacterial endocarditis, and anaerobic streptococci play an important part in surgical and puerperal sepsis.

Infection with *Strep. pyogenes* is common in temperate zones and has its highest incidence in children during winter. The infection is often symptomless, with up to 20% of children carrying the organism in their throat. The source of human infection may be a carrier or a patient suffering from streptococcal disease, especially of the upper respiratory tract. Children are more likely to transmit infection than adults. Convalescent carriers are more infectious than chronic carriers; nasal carriers are less common than pharyngeal carriers but shed large numbers of organisms and are more dangerous.

Infection is usually spread by droplets of secretions sprayed from the air passages by sneezing, spluttering, or coughing; the organism may also be transmitted indirectly by hand contact, dust, or fomites. Outbreaks of tonsillitis or scarlet fever may originate from contaminated foodstuffs, including milk.

The outcome of streptococcal infections depends on the virulence of the organism and the resistance of the host. If antibacterial immunity is high the streptococcus may fail to become established or may be confined to the surface of the mucosa or skin of the host; if antibacterial resistance is low or if the streptococcus is highly virulent surface invasion may result in tonsillitis or impetigo, and deeper penetration may lead to lymphadenitis or septicaemia. If the invading organism produces large amounts of erythrogenic toxin, and antitoxic immunity is also low, then scarlet fever results.

Organism

1   Smear of pus showing streptococci (Gram stain). Streptococci are Gram-positive, spherical or oval cells, measuring 0.5–0.75µm in diameter, and are arranged in pairs or chains of varying lengths. They are non-motile and do not form spores. Capsules may be seen in young cultures but are not prominent; most are aerobes or facultative anaerobes, but some are anaerobic or microaerophilic.

2   Blood agar culture showing beta-haemolysis. Some aerobic streptococci produce a soluble haemolysin which creates a clear zone of haemolysis on fresh blood agar. This is termed beta-haemolysis. Colonies are less than 1 mm in diameter and are surrounded by a clear colourless zone within which the red cells are completely haemolysed. Haemolysis is striking when *Strep. pyogenes* is cultured anaerobically and may occasionally be absent on aerobic culture.

Surface infections

Streptococcal infections of the upper respiratory tract

3   Appearance of the lips and mouth in streptococcal tonsillitis. Streptococcal infection of the throat is commonly accompanied by changes in the appearance of the lips, which become glazed and cherry-red in hue. Moist cracks may be found at the corners of the mouth.

4   Cervical lymphadenitis. Infection may spread from the tonsils to the cervical lymph nodes, causing suppurative lymphadenitis. In young children the swelling of the neck may be disproportionate to the degree of inflammation in the throat and may be confused with mumps. However, careful examination will distinguish lymph node swelling from that of the salivary glands.

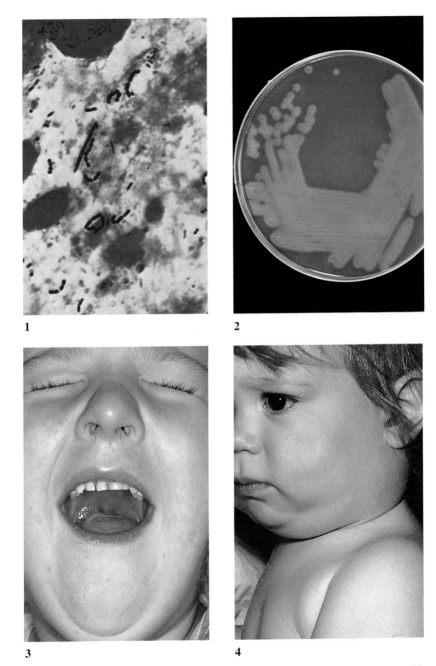

5   Inflamed tonsils without exudate. The appearance of the throat may be identical in both viral and streptococcal infections, so it is difficult without laboratory tests to be certain about the aetiology of mild tonsillitis. In the illustration redness and congestion extend across the arch of the palate to the oedematous uvula.

In infants and children under 3 years the focal signs of tonsillitis are less prominent and exudate is seldom present. If untreated the illness tends to follow a prolonged course with low-grade fever. Vomiting and abdominal pain may confuse the clinical picture.

6   Inflamed tonsils with exudate. In older children and adults the onset is more abrupt, with a painful throat accompanied by general disturbance with fever, headache and malaise. The fauces are inflamed, the tonsils swollen, and patches of white or yellow exudate are present in about half of patients. The tonsillar lymph nodes become enlarged and tender. In this group of patients the illness is of short duration.

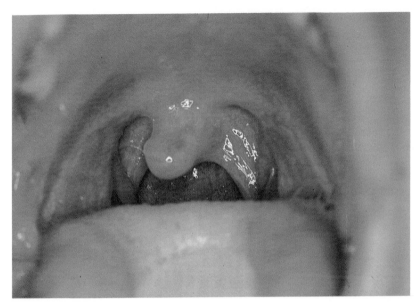

5

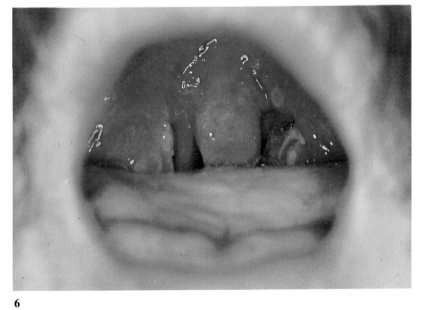

6

7   Follicular tonsillitis. The degree of congestion varies considerably, and follicular exudate may be present on the tonsils with minimal reaction in the surrounding tissues.

8   Peritonsillar abscess (quinsy). When a streptococcus spreads from the tonsil into the adjacent soft tissues congestion and swelling increase rapidly, and suppuration usually follows. Patients experience great difficulty in opening their mouth, swallowing becomes exquisitely painful and the voice develops a nasal intonation. The anterior wall of the fauces bulges and displaces the uvula to the opposite side. Pus forms and tracks to the surface, where it points as a yellow spot through which it eventually discharges. If antibiotic treatment is given at an early stage, the infection is usually brought under control before an abscess forms and the cellulitis subsides uneventfully.

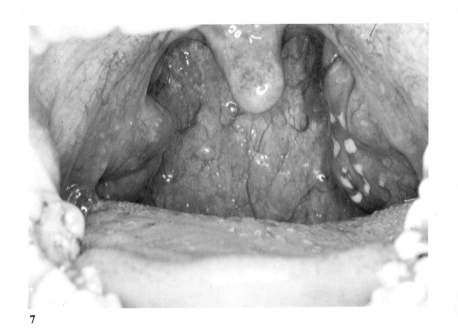

7

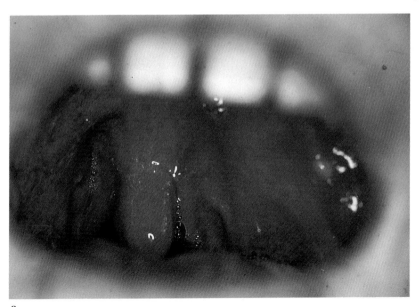

8

15

9   Ludwig's angina – front view. Ludwig's angina is the term applied to a severe form of cellulitis in the region of the submandibular gland. It is usually caused by spread of infection to the connective tissue planes from a suppurating lymph node, secondary to tonsillitis or dental infection. A streptococcus is usually responsible, although there may be a mixed infection with anaerobes.

10   Ludwig's angina – side view.

11   Ludwig's angina – floor of mouth. Inflammatory oedema distorts the floor of the mouth and makes swallowing difficult. Oedema of the glottis may arise suddenly and cause dangerous respiratory obstruction.

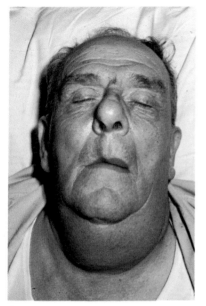

9

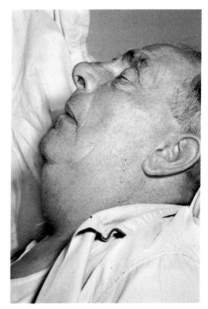

10

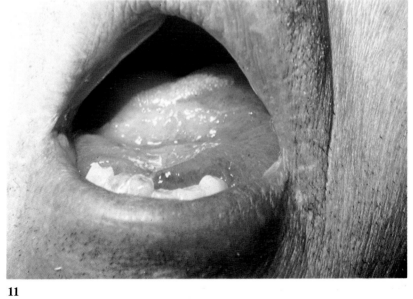

11

Scarlet fever

12   Circumoral pallor and rash on trunk. Scarlet fever is caused by an erythrogenic strain of *Strep. pyogenes* invading a susceptible host. The portal of entry is usually the throat, but scarlet fever may follow infection of a wound, burn, or other skin lesion, such as a chickenpox vesicle. This type of scarlet fever with infection of the skin is commonly designated 'surgical scarlet fever'. Infection of the genital tract during childbirth may give rise to 'puerperal scarlet fever'.

The onset of scarlet fever is sudden, with a sharp febrile reaction, soreness of the throat, and vomiting. In a mild attack vomiting may be absent and some children may not complain of a sore throat. The exanthem follows within 24–36 hours and evolves from above downwards. There is a bright flush on the cheeks and chin, which contrasts vividly with the pallor around the mouth. Elsewhere there is an erythematous background of varying intensity with tiny superficial red spots or puncta. This punctate erythema is most prominent over the neck and upper chest. Over the distal part of the limbs the rash may condense into discrete macules. Pallor around the mouth is seen in other conditions, especially lobar pneumonia.

Complications of scarlet fever fall into two categories: septic (consisting of rhinitis, sinusitis, otitis media, and suppurative lymphadenitis); and immunological (consisting of rheumatic fever and nephritis).

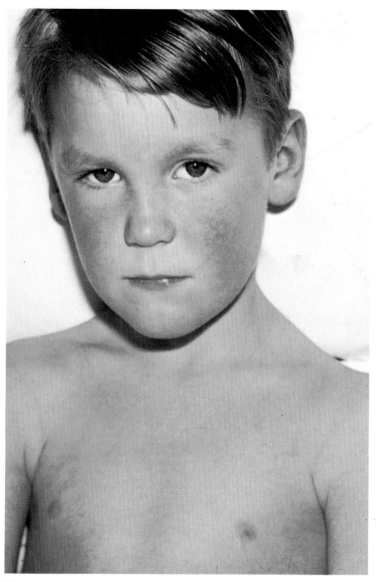

12

13   Punctate erythema on trunk. The punctate erythematous rash is most prominent over the neck and upper chest, where it resembles flushed gooseflesh.

14   Rash on thigh. The rash on the limbs is blotchy and may coalesce into discrete macules distally. It may be difficult to distinguish the rash of scarlet fever from that of rubella, but the characteristic appearance of the mouth and throat in scarlet fever will indicate the correct diagnosis.

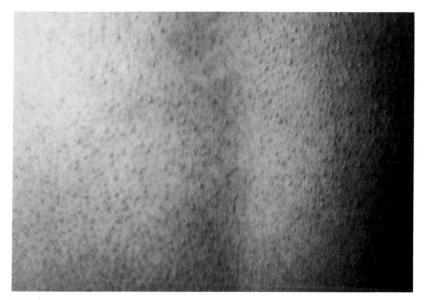

13

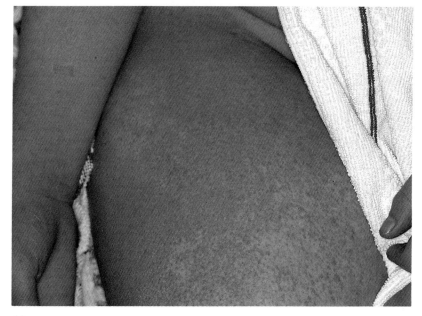

14

15 **'Surgical scarlet fever' from an infected cut.** Absorption of erythrogenic toxin from an infected wound or skin lesion gives rise to scarlet fever in a susceptible person. The typical enanthem is present even when the streptococcus is confined to the skin lesion (see also scarlet fever in chickenpox – **231** and **232**).

16 **Pastia's sign.** Petechiae may be found in the antecubital fossa when the rash is heavy. After the erythema fades the pigmentation persists and is described as Pastia's sign, now mainly of historical interest.

17 **Desquamation on the hand.** About 4–5 days after onset of the rash the skin begins to peel. Small patches of desquamation appear on the neck and thorax and spread downwards to the hands and feet by the end of the second week. The amount of peeling varies greatly but tends to be pronounced when the erythema has been intense. After the rash has faded desquamation is a helpful diagnostic clue but is not pathognomonic of scarlet fever. Desquamation begins with a minute central pinhole surrounded by a small collar of epidermis which separates to form flakes.

18 **Desquamation on the hand.** Towards the end of the second week the skin splits round the nail folds, and coarse strips may peel from the thick skin of the hands and feet.

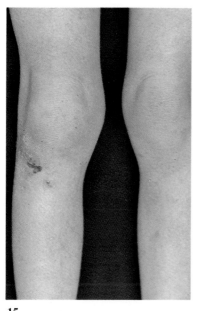

15

16

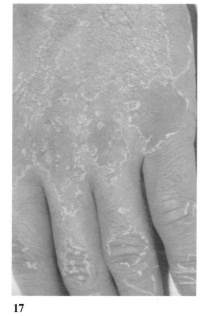

17

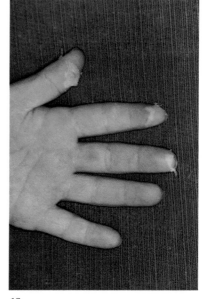

18

19 White strawberry tongue. During the first day or two the tongue is covered with a thick white fur through which the enlarged red papillae protrude. The palate is stippled with dark red macules and occasionally a few petechiae. The fauces are vividly red and swollen, and there may be patches of white exudate on the tonsils.

20 Red strawberry tongue. Within a few days the fur peels from the tip and edges of the tongue to produce the red strawberry stage. The illustration shows the red, glazed surface with prominent papillae and the remnants of white fur.

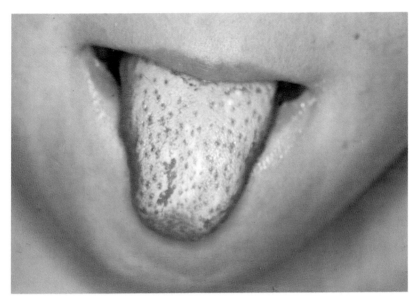

19

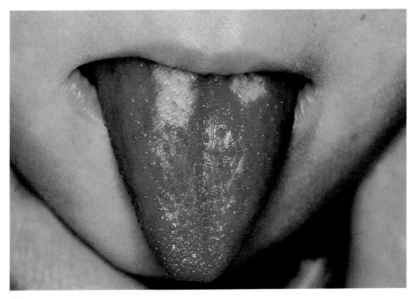

20

Erysipelas

21   Butterfly-wing rash on the face. Erysipelas is often preceded by an upper respiratory infection and is more common in older age groups with degenerative skin changes which allow easy penetration by the streptococcus. It usually affects the face or legs, and infection may possibly be transferred on the patient's fingers to these 'scratch areas' of the body. The streptococcus generally invades through an invisible breach in the skin and spreads centrifugally from the point of entry through the lymphatics. Infection may be confined to the skin or extend into the subcutaneous tissues. Occasionally the streptococcus may gain access through a surgical wound, leg ulcer, or the umbilical stump in a newborn infant.

After a short incubation period of less than a week, the illness starts abruptly with general symptoms. Within a few hours an unpleasant sensation of tightness and burning develops at the site of invasion, followed quickly by a patch of erythema which rapidly extends outwards. The spreading edge is sharply defined as a palpable ridge. Bullae may form in the central erythematous zone and rupture, leaving raw weeping areas.

Erysipelas of the face often starts on one cheek and spreads across the nose to the other side producing a characteristic butterfly-wing appearance. Occasionally it may be confined to one side.

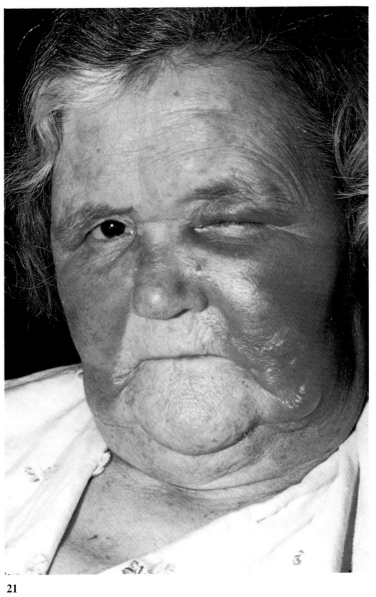

21

22   Erysipelas of the face – acute stage. During the acute stage the eyelids may become so swollen that they cannot be opened, and the eyelashes may be matted by purulent discharge. This is commonly confused with herpes ophthalmicus, but the hemicranial distribution of herpes should prevent error (see **247**).

23   Erysipelas of the face – convalescent stage. Once infection has been overcome the inflammation subsides, leaving pigmentation and desquamation in the affected area. For some months afterwards exposure to cold wind or strong sunshine may cause local flushing.

24   Erysipelas of the leg – acute stage. Infection may spread into the subcutaneous tissues to produce an erysipelo-cellulitis. Bullae are common and may rupture with discharge of seropurulent fluid. Necrosis sometimes occurs.

25   Erysipelas of the leg – convalescent stage. Pigmentation and desquamation are prominent features. Damage to lymph vessels may obstruct lymphatic flow and cause persistent oedema, which predisposes the patient to further attacks.

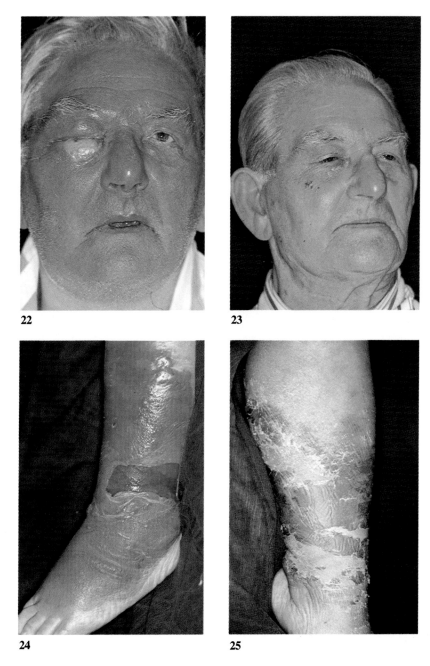

22

23

24

25

Impetigo

26   Impetigo contagiosa of the face. Impetigo is a highly contagious superficial infection of the skin caused either by streptococci or by staphylococci. The disease may affect an apparently normal skin or complicate some underlying skin condition, such as pediculosis, scabies, eczema, or acute fungus infection. It commonly starts on the face around the mouth or nose, spreading with alarming rapidity to other parts of the body. In streptococcal impetigo the exudate dries to form a thick crust with a golden yellow colour. (Contrast with staphylococcal impetigo: **44–46**.)

27   Impetigo contagiosa of the leg. The thick crusts protect the underlying streptococci from local applications. Skin infection with nephritogenic strains of streptococci may cause outbreaks of acute nephritis.

Invasion of deeper tissues

Cellulitis

28   Cellulitis. When a streptococcus enters through a breach in the skin or mucosa it may provoke a local reaction of cellulitis, may spread into the lymph vessels, giving rise to lymphangitis and lymphadenitis, or may invade the bloodstream, causing septicaemia. The zone of inflammation is less sharply demarcated in cellulitis than in erysipelas, and is frequently followed by suppuration.

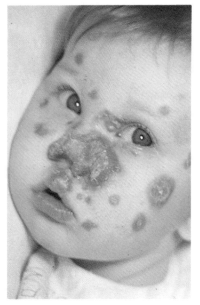

26

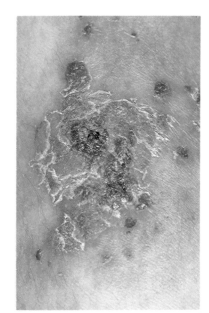

27

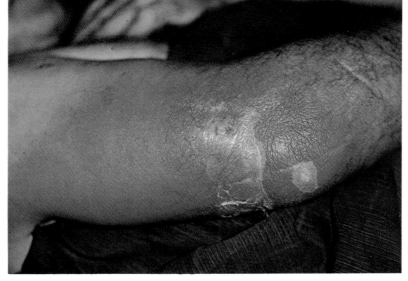

28

Septicaemia

29   Septicaemia. Invasion of the bloodstream by *Strep. pyogenes* may produce metastatic lesions with haemorrhages and focal cellulitis. The local reaction is overshadowed by the general disturbance.

30   Brain abscess. Streptococci of low virulence, entering the bloodstream in small numbers, produce minimal general disturbance but may lodge in an organ such as the brain, causing local damage and abscesses. These streptococci are usually microaerophilic or anaerobic. There may be a long interval before clinical signs appear.

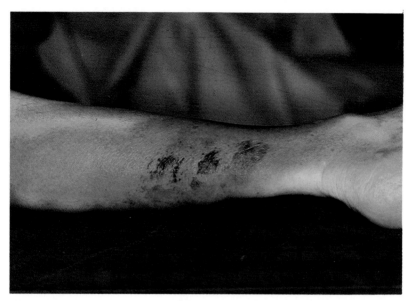

29

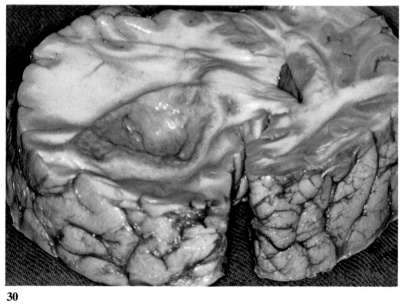

30

31   Subacute bacterial endocarditis. Most streptococcal infections in humans are caused by beta-haemolytic strains, but other streptococci may be responsible for serious disease. Viridans streptococci, normal inhabitants of the mouth, may gain access to the bloodstream through the teeth or gums and cause endocarditis, particularly if a heart valve is already defective. The illness manifests as an unexplained fever, which can be diagnosed with certainty during life only when the organism is recovered from blood cultures, although the echocardiographic appearances can be highly suggestive.

The vegetations formed on the heart valves are larger, softer, and more crumbling in character than those found in rheumatic heart disease, and tend to spread on the endocardial surface. Destruction of the valves is less than in acute bacterial endocarditis. The small emboli, thrown from the outer layer of the vegetation, seldom contain organisms and therefore cause bland infarcts. A high proportion terminate in the kidneys and brain. The arrows on the figure indicate vegetations.

32   Subacute bacterial endocarditis – histology of heart valve. The vegetation has three layers. The outer layer or cap has an eosinophilic granular appearance and consists of platelets in a matrix of fibrin. Streptococci occupy the middle zone, and the base is formed by the inflamed cusp. Most small emboli, so common in subacute bacterial endocarditis, are shed from the outer layer. (A = myocardium, B = cusp, C = cap.)

33   Subacute bacterial endocarditis – splinter haemorrhages. Deposition of immune complexes may give rise to petechial haemorrhages in the conjunctivas, buccal mucosa or skin, or to linear haemorrhages under the nails. Small tender nodules (Osler's nodes) may be found in the pulps of the fingers or toes. Glomerulonephritis is common.

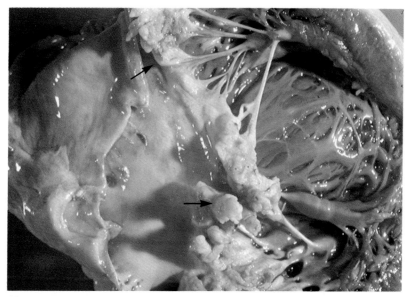

31

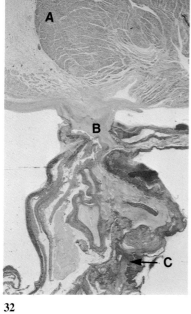

32

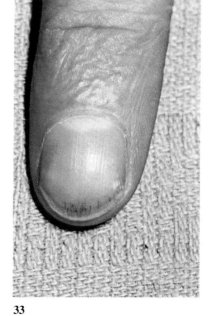

33

Sensitisation reactions to streptococci

34   Erythema nodosum – distribution of rash. The rash of erythema nodosum consists of tender nodules, ranging in diameter from 1 to 5 cm. The eruption is prominent over the shins but may also be present on the arms or face. The condition is found mainly in young adults and may follow sensitisation to a number of agents including beta-haemolytic streptococci. Constitutional disturbance is variable; fever is often present and lymph nodes may be enlarged.

35   Erythema nodosum – rash on legs. During the acute stage the nodules are red and painful; as the rash subsides the nodules pass through the range of colours seen in a fading bruise. The nodules never ulcerate, and there is no residual scarring.

36   Erythema marginatum. Erythema marginatum, also known as rheumatic erythema, is a circinate erythema resulting from streptococcal sensitisation. This fluctuating rash is found mainly in children and is most prominent on the trunk. It is sometimes associated with subacute rheumatic fever.

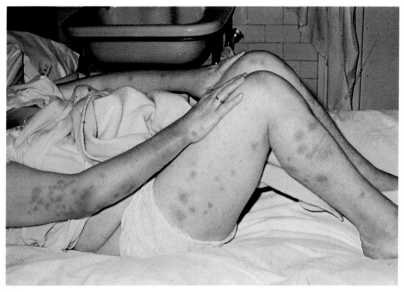

34

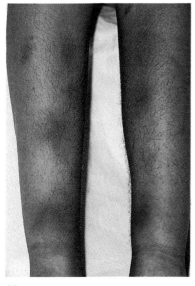

35

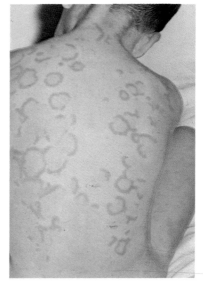

36

37

Staphylococcal infection

Staphylococci are widely distributed in nature. Many are saprophytic and can be isolated from water and soil; others are parasitic and may be found as commensals or pathogens in humans or animals. Two species are of medical importance – *Staphylococcus aureus* and the less virulent *Staphylococcus epidermidis*.

Staph. aureus is a common organism on the skin of humans and animals in all parts of the world. The sites most heavily colonised in humans are the nasal vestibule, the perineum, groin, axilla, and umbilicus. The organism is present in the anterior nares of 36–50% of normal adults; the nasal carriage rate in hospital patients may be as high as 70%. The source of infection is usually a human and staphylococci may be spread by autoinfection, by direct or indirect contact with an asymptomatic carrier harbouring the organism in the anterior nares or other site, or may be derived from a patient with a discharging staphylococcal lesion.

Staph. epidermidis, formerly regarded as a non-pathogenic commensal of the skin, gives rise to infection in hospitals, particularly in immunocompromised patients and those with a prosthesis such as a cardiac valve, vascular cannula, or cerebrospinal fluid shunt.

Organism

37   Smear of pus containing staphylococci (Gram stain). Staphylococci are Gram-positive, spherical cocci measuring roughly 1 μm in diameter. They are grouped in clusters resembling bunches of grapes, but single forms and pairs may also be found.

38   *Staph. aureus* – culture on blood agar. *Staph. aureus* is a facultative anaerobe, which grows readily on blood agar forming relatively large colonies, with a diameter of 2–4 mm after 24 hours. Mature colonies are opaque, convex, circular discs with a shiny surface and golden colour. Zones of haemolysis appear on sheep or rabbit blood agar; haemolysis is minimal or absent on horse blood agar.

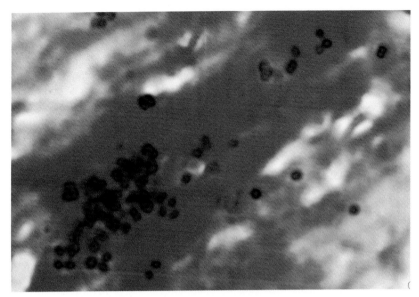

37

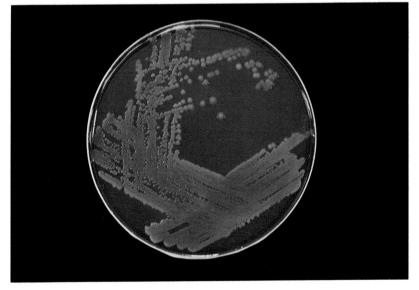

38

39   Coagulase test. Pathogenic strains of staphylococci may be identified by their ability to clot blood plasma. The production of coagulase is probably the most reliable *in vitro* guide to pathogenicity: DNAse production may also be helpful in identifying *Staph. aureus*. Many other toxins are elaborated by staphylococci but little is known of their part in producing disease. Some strains of *Staph. aureus* produce an enterotoxin responsible for outbreaks of food poisoning; others produce toxins responsible for scalded-skin and staphylococcal-shock syndromes.

In the two tubes of plasma shown in the illustration the control has remained fluid, while that inoculated with *Staph. aureus* has clotted.

40   Phage typing – typical pattern using standard phages. Bacteriophages are viruses capable of growing in bacterial cells and causing them to lyse. Most strains of *Staph. aureus* may be destroyed by several bacteriophages; some strains are untypable. Using a combination of typing phages several hundred strains have been identified, and phage typing has proved a useful epidemiological tool.

Drops containing each of the typing phages have been placed in a prescribed pattern on the surface of the medium after it has been evenly inoculated with the staphylococcus. Lysis has taken place where the bacteria have been attacked by particular phages. Staphylococci may be allotted to four groups by the pattern of lysis. Those in groups I and III are associated with hospital sepsis. Virulent epidemic strains of *Staph. aureus* may emerge in hospitals as a result of the unrestricted use of antibiotics and some are highly resistant to treatment. These resistant strains have been designated MRSA (methicillin resistant *Staphylococcus aureus*).

Staphylococcal infection of the skin

Staphylococcal skin disease is endemic throughout the world. It is most common in warm climates, particularly in children in overcrowded, unhygienic conditions.

41   Stye (hordeolum). Staphylococcal invasion of a hair follicle gives rise to a small abscess or boil. When this affects the sebaceous gland of an eyelash follicle the resulting abscess is called a stye or hordeolum. The term 'furunculosis' is applied to recurring crops of boils. Diabetes mellitus is an important, though uncommon, predisposing factor in furunculosis.

42   Carbuncle. When several adjacent hair follicles are affected the abscesses merge to form a carbuncle. The central necrotic core sloughs, leaving a large ulcer and disfiguring scar. The possibility of underlying diabetes mellitus should always be borne in mind.

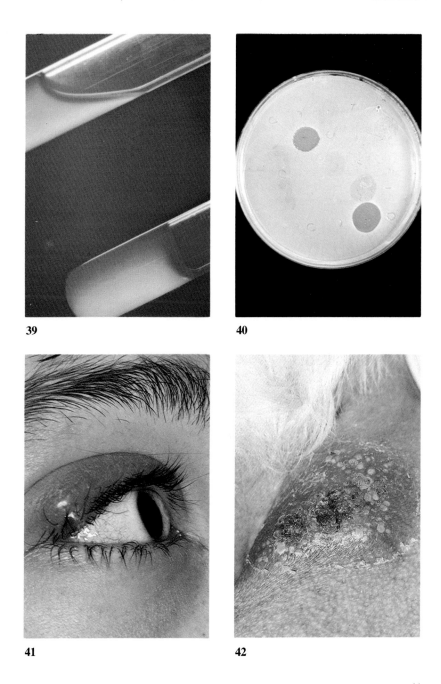

39

40

41

42

43 Histology of skin abscess (haematoxylin and eosin stain). Local invasion of the skin is rapidly followed by an inflammatory reaction, with infiltration of pus cells and the formation of a sharply demarcated abscess. The outer wall consists of a layer of fibroblasts, providing an effective barrier to the spread of staphylococci unless ruptured by squeezing or surgery. Tension within the abscess may increase as the central core liquefies and the abscess may rupture spontaneously on the surface of the body; occasionally infection may spread to surrounding tissues.

Coagulase-positive staphylococci are readily engulfed by phagocytes. They are able to survive inside the phagocytes, and even multiply before ultimately destroying the phagocytes and escaping. Antibody production does not seem to play an important part in preventing infection.

Note the striking contrast between staphylococcal infection, where the inflammatory reaction extends into the subcutaneous tissues, and viral infections (such as varicella), where the changes are confined to the epidermis (see **216–17**). The arrow indicates the junction of the dermis with subcutaneous tissue.

44 Bullous impetigo of the face. Superficial infection of the skin with *Staph. aureus* causes one variety of impetigo (see **26**). The rash usually begins around the nose or mouth and spreads rapidly to other parts of the body. Staphylococcal impetigo may take the form of bullae, containing pus, which rupture and produce crusts.

Staphylococcal impetigo is highly infectious in infants and young children; death may result from systemic invasion.

45 Pustular impetigo. In older patients pustular lesions predominate and systemic spread is rare. Phage group II staphylococci are commonly involved and many are resistant to benzylpenicillin.

46 Crusted impetigo. Bullae dry up and usually become crusted within a few hours; occasionally crusts may form after a delay of a day or two. Staphylococcal crusts do not have the golden-yellow hue of streptococcal lesions (see **26**).

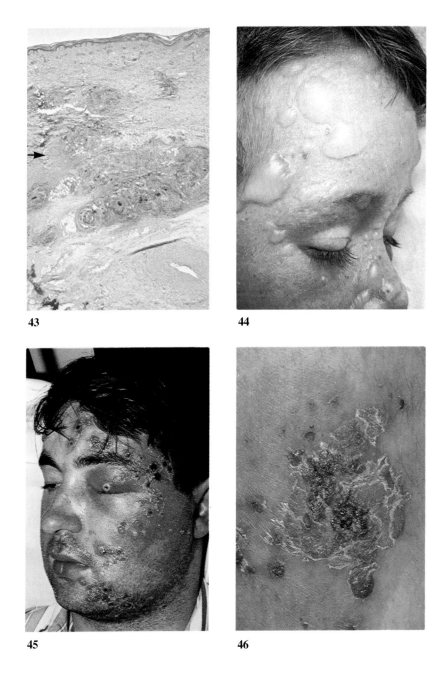

47   Scalded-skin syndrome (acute epidermal necrolysis; Lyell's syndrome). Scalded-skin syndrome closely resembles Stevens–Johnson syndrome. Both conditions are characterised by conjunctivitis, stomatitis, urethritis, and a rash. However, the skin lesions are different. In scalded-skin syndrome the skin is extremely painful and large patches of necrotic epidermis slide off the underlying layers at the slightest pressure leaving extensive raw areas (Nikolsky's sign). The appearance closely resembles a severe scald.

There appear to be two varieties of scalded-skin syndrome: one associated with group II staphylococci (especially phage-type 71), the other with hypersensitivity to drugs. In the infectious variety staphylococci growing on the surface of the skin or mucosae produce an epidermolytic exotoxin, exfoliatin, that damages the skin cells, resulting in cleavage within the epidermis at the level of the stratum granulosum (see **494–8**).

48   Ritter's disease. Ritter's disease appears to be a neonatal form of scalded-skin syndrome. The illness begins abruptly with redness and crusting round the mouth followed within a day or two by a generalised erythematous rash. The skin is painful and flaccid bullae develop. The slightest pressure rubs away the surface of the skin, leaving raw areas. During the acute stage systemic disturbance with fever occurs. Mucous membranes are seldom affected. After several days the erythema begins to subside and is followed by desquamation. The skin is restored to normal within 7–10 days. Systemic invasion may occasionally lead to death.

Toxic-shock syndrome

49   Rash. Most cases of toxic-shock syndrome have been associated with the use of tampons during menstruation; some have followed staphylococcal infection at other sites. *Staph. aureus* in the vagina elaborates enterotoxin F, which is absorbed and produces widespread tissue damage. The illness is characterised by fever, an erythematous rash appearing simultaneously on all parts of the body, diarrhoea, myalgia accompanied by high blood levels of creatinine phosphokinase, tachycardia, and hypotension. The illness is severe and may be life-threatening. The rash has no characteristic features.

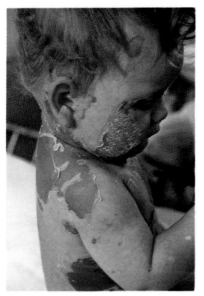

47

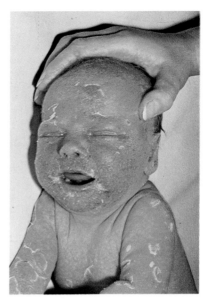

48

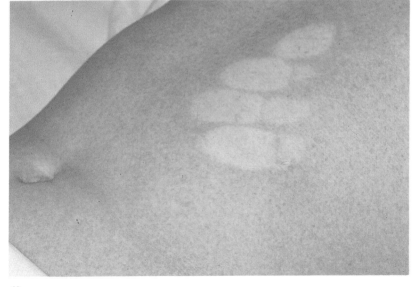

49

Staphylococcal septicaemia

Severe staphylococcal disease may be found in highly susceptible persons, such as the elderly following influenza, intravenous drug abusers, and debilitated or immunocompromised patients in hospitals. Wound infections are a frequent manifestation of hospital-acquired staphylococci.

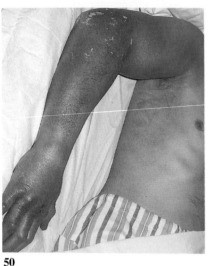

50 Cellulitis of upper limb and chest wall in septicaemia. Local infection of the soft tissues with *Staph. aureus* will produce cellulitis, and subsequent spread into the bloodstream gives rise to septicaemia. Occasionally metastatic infection from a septicaemia may cause cellulitis.

50

51 Haemorrhages under nails. In many cases of staphylococcal septicaemia there is no obvious portal of entry; in others septicaemia may follow sepsis in the skin or genital tract. In the early stages general symptoms dominate. If the patient survives, metastatic abscesses usually appear. Toxic damage to capillary endothelium or multiple emboli from acute endocarditis cause bleeding into the skin and under the nails. The lesions are more florid than those seen in subacute endocarditis (see **33**). Blood cultures must be taken and sensitivity tests performed on any isolates.

52 Haemorrhages into toes. Skin haemorrhages are found in many types of septicaemia but are particularly common in staphylococcal and meningococcal infection.

53 Gangrene of feet. Massive emboli or arterial thrombosis may complicate overwhelming infection, especially in elderly or debilitated patients.

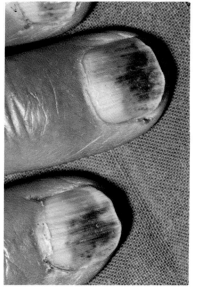

51

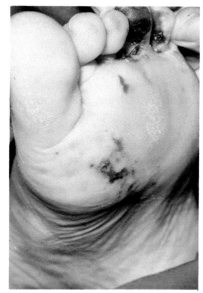

52

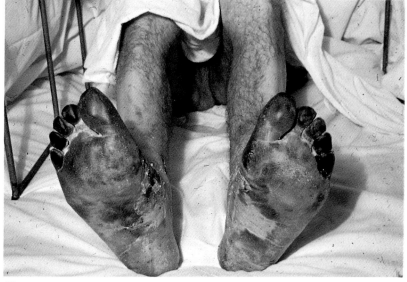

53

Staphylococcal scarlet fever

54   Septic hand. Some strains of staphylococci apparently produce an erythro-genic toxin, which gives rise to the clinical picture of scarlet fever.

A pure culture of *Staph. aureus* was obtained from the septic lesions on this patient's hand. Throat and hand swabs yielded negative results for haemolytic streptococci, and the antistreptolysin O titre failed to rise.

55   Rash – close-up. The rash closely resembles that seen in streptococcal scarlet fever, but the puncta are not so pronounced. Desquamation follows.

56   Appearance of the tongue. In the early stages of both staphylococcal and streptococcal scarlet fever there is circumoral pallor and a white strawberry tongue (see **19**). Subsequently the fur peels leaving a typical red strawberry appearance.

Puerperal sepsis

57   Puerperal sepsis – staphylococcal mastitis. If an epidemic strain of staphylococcus is introduced into a maternity unit the brunt of the attack is borne by the babies. The cycle is continued from baby to baby with the older ones forming the reservoir of infection. The baby's nose is rapidly colonised and over 90% may be infected by the time of discharge. The sepsis rate among the neonates is generally 10–20%. Most of the infections are trivial, consisting of pustules and septic bullae, particularly around the nail folds, but occasionally the consequences are more serious, with invasion of the deeper tissues.

In nursing mothers staphylococci derived from the baby may invade the breast, causing mastitis with suppuration. These breast abscesses commonly develop 6–8 weeks after delivery and may be the first indication of a staphylo-coccal outbreak in a maternity unit. Note the superficial pustules on the skin around the inflamed breast.

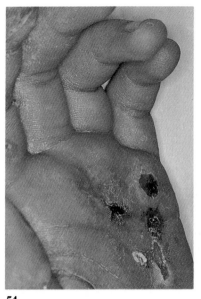

54

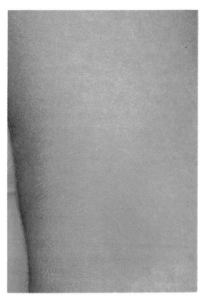

55

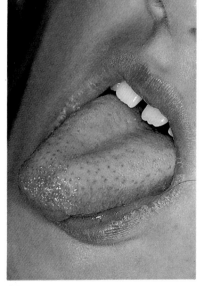

56

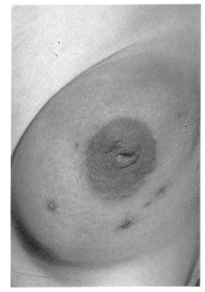

57

49

Osteomyelitis

58   Osteomyelitis – radiograph of tibia. The bloodstream may be invaded from a focal lesion on the skin or nasopharynx, although in many cases there is no obvious portal of entry. In children with septicaemia, staphylococci may lodge in the metaphysis of a long bone producing osteomyelitis, especially following a recent trivial injury to a limb. Initially the illness is dominated by toxaemia with high fever and delirium; later the affected bone becomes acutely tender and the slightest movement causes severe distress. During the early septicaemic phase the white blood cell count is frequently normal or even depressed, but as infection localises in bone a polymorphonuclear leucocytosis develops. Changes are not usually detectable on radiographic examination until 2–3 weeks have elapsed, but bone scans are frequently suggestive of the diagnosis at the time of initial presentation.

Patchy decalcification and periosteal reaction with deposition of new bone are the characteristic findings. In untreated cases infection spreading to the periosteum and rising pressure within the medullary cavity may interfere with the blood supply, causing necrosis of bone. Eventually a balance is reached between the formation of new bone and the destruction of old. In chronic osteomyelitis the anti-staphylolysin titre may be raised.

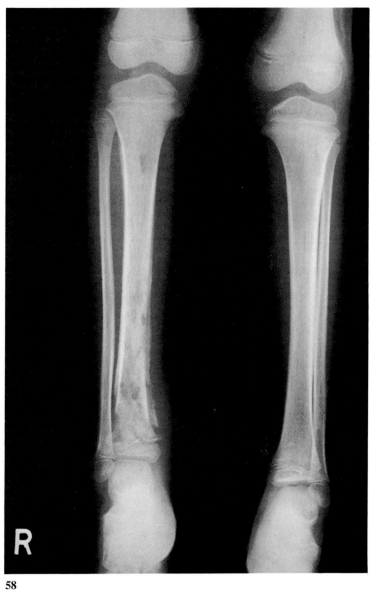

R

58

Pneumonia

59 **Staphylococcal pneumonia – chest radiograph.** Staphylococcal pneumonia may complicate influenza and other viral infections, especially in patients with chronic bronchitis or uraemia. It may also follow surgical treatment or result from an outbreak of sepsis in a maternity unit. Invasion of the lungs from the upper respiratory passages may produce tracheobronchitis, bronchopneumonia, or multiple abscesses. Staphylococcal infection damages the walls of the smaller bronchi, which may rupture, allowing air to escape into the interstitial tissues. Air then accumulates under tension as a result of a ball-valve action and the typical pneumatoceles of severe staphylococcal pneumonia are formed. Rupture of a lung abscess into the pleural cavity produces an empyema or pyopneumothorax.

The radiograph of the child's chest shows collapse of the lung on the right and marked displacement of the mediastinum to the left as a result of pyopneumothorax on the right side. Staphylococcal pus was aspirated from the pleural cavity (see **233**).

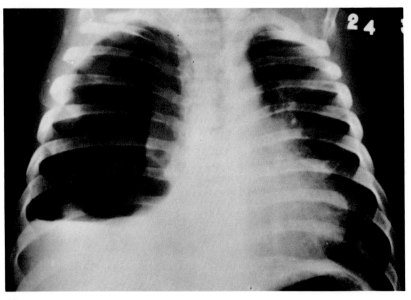

59

Meningococcal infection

Acute meningitis is an inflammation of the membranes surrounding the brain and spinal cord. A great variety of micro-organisms, varying in complexity from viruses to protozoa, have been found in patients with meningitis; however, for clinical purposes the disease may be classified simply into aseptic and pyogenic forms. Acute pyogenic meningitis is caused by a wide range of bacteria, the most common being the meningococcus, *Haemophilus influenzae*, and the pneumococcus. Enterobacteria (principally *Escherichia coli*), group B streptococci, *Staph. aureus*, and *Listeria monocytogenes* are found more commonly in neonates than other age groups. *Staph. epidermidis* is particularly associated with pressure-relieving valves in hydrocephalus; anaerobes are rarely isolated.

The meningococcus is a human parasite closely related to the gonococcus (see **180**) and has a worldwide distribution. The highest incidence of infection is in preschool children, although it is common in older children and young adults. Usually about 50% of cases are under 5 years of age but the proportion in older children and young adults may rise during epidemics. Outbreaks may occur in schools and other closed or semi-closed communities, where susceptible people congregate. Community outbreaks appear periodically, notably in sub-Saharan Africa, where annual epidemics take place in spring and especially affect the poorer classes.

Nasopharyngeal carriage is common and its duration varies with the strain; the overall prevalence is usually 2–4% of the population but may rise to 20% in epidemics and may exceed 50% if outbreaks involve enclosed communities. In most individuals the meningococcus remains confined to the nasopharynx, where there is little or no reaction, but it occasionally invades the bloodstream or spreads to the meninges with disastrous consequences. Factors leading to the development of disease are not known but may be associated with secretory immunoglobulin (IgA) deficiency on mucosal cells, with passive smoking, or with intercurrent respiratory infections.

Organism and pathology

N. meningitidis can be divided into eight serotypes according to the nature of the cell-wall polysaccharides, namely, A, B, C, X, Y (or Bo), Z, 135 and 29E. Some are 'untypable'. Groups A, B and C are traditionally associated with outbreaks of disease while other types are common in carriers. Group A strains are common in Africa, the Arabian peninsula, northern India and Nepal; groups A and C in Brazil; groups B and C in North America and Europe.

60 Smear of purulent cerebrospinal fluid showing meningococcus (Gram stain). *Neisseria meningitidis* is a fastidious Gram-negative diplococcus with flattened adjacent sides. It has no demonstrable capsule. The organism is frequently present within cells in cerebrospinal fluid from patients with meningococcal meningitis. It is an aerobe and primary cultures are obtained most readily on enriched media, such as chocolate blood agar, in an atmosphere containing 10% carbon dioxide. *N. meningitidis* is identified biochemically or by immunofluorescence.

61 Purulent cerebrospinal fluid. Meningococci are disseminated in droplets from the upper respiratory tract, the usual source being an unsuspected carrier.

A diagnosis of pyogenic meningitis is established by finding turbid cerebrospinal fluid on lumbar puncture. The nature of the infection may be suspected by the abruptness of onset of the illness in a young person, or by the presence of a haemorrhagic rash, and the diagnosis confirmed by the detection of Gram-negative intracellular diplococci in a smear of cerebrospinal fluid. Meningococci may be cultured from cerebrospinal fluid or blood.

62 Appearance of the brain and meninges. It is commonly believed that the meningococcus spreads to the meninges via the bloodstream but direct spread from the nasopharynx has not been completely excluded.

Once the meninges have been invaded there is an acute inflammatory reaction with congestion and oedema, petechial haemorrhages and marked distension of the veins. Within 48 hours a thin layer of pus covers the brain, especially round the base, and the ventricles become distended with turbid fluid. The foramina may become blocked with viscous fluid and adhesions may further impair the free flow of cerebrospinal fluid.

Although the disease is essentially a leptomeningitis, changes are also found in the substance of the brain, where there is swelling, vascular engorgement, and toxic damage to nerve cells.

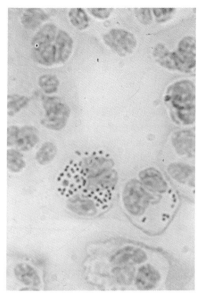

60

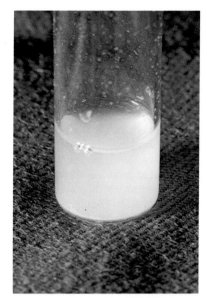

61

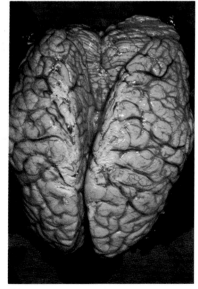

62

Clinical features

63   Meningitis – neck stiffness and head retraction. The onset of meningococcal meningitis in older children and adults is usually sudden, with violent headache, feverishness and vomiting as the presenting symptoms. In the early stages of the illness it may be possible to flex the neck but stiffness quickly develops and the manoeuvre causes great discomfort.

Neck stiffness is a feature of all forms of meningeal irritation and is found in such diverse conditions as meningitis, brain abscesses, tumours, subarachnoid haemorrhage, and meningismus associated with infection of the respiratory passages or renal tract. In children under the age of 2 years the presenting features of meningitis are very variable and neck stiffness is seldom marked.

This patient was highly irritable and preferred to lie undisturbed on his side with his back to the light. Minor degrees of head retraction are common, although the advanced state of opisthotonus is seldom seen when treatment is effective. Increasing drowsiness, sometimes accompanied by convulsions, leads to coma.

64   Early rash. The incidence of rashes in patients with meningococcal meningitis varies considerably: during epidemics it may be as high as 50%, but in sporadic cases it rarely exceeds 20%. Fleeting macular or papular rashes are not uncommon in young children in the early septicaemic stage of the disease. In some cases the rash progresses no further; in others the rash alters, with the development of bleeding into the skin and mucous membranes. Some patients die in the septicaemic stage of the illness; most (90%) progress rapidly to acute meningitis. In this child the haemorrhages are just beginning to appear in the erythematous lesions. The rash quickly became haemorrhagic and consisted of petechiae and small ecchymoses. The combination of purulent cerebrospinal fluid and a haemorrhagic rash is almost diagnostic of meningococcal meningitis.

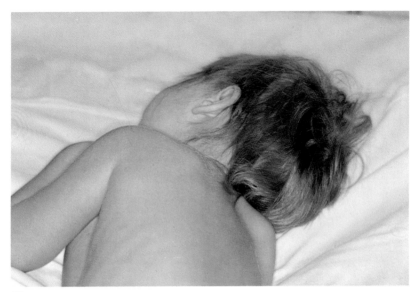

63

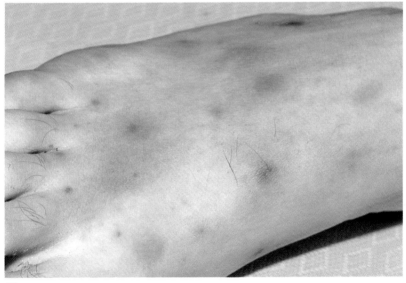

64

65   Meningitis – unconscious patient with rash. This child was admitted to hospital unconscious and found to have a sparse rash with petechiae and small ecchymoses. *N. meningitidis* was grown on from blood and from the purulent cerebrospinal fluid. Response to treatment was good and recovery was uneventful.

66   Meningitis – haemorrhagic rash in a young child. In very young children the onset of meningitis may be so insidious that the possibility may be overlooked for several days. Unexplained fever or vomiting, with or without diarrhoea, should always arouse suspicion of meningitis. Neck stiffness may be absent, but there is often some fullness of the anterior fontanelle. Convulsions occur in about a third of children with purulent meningitis, but are common in other infections. The incidence of meningococcal meningitis is less in this age group, but the disease should be suspected whenever there is a haemorrhagic rash.

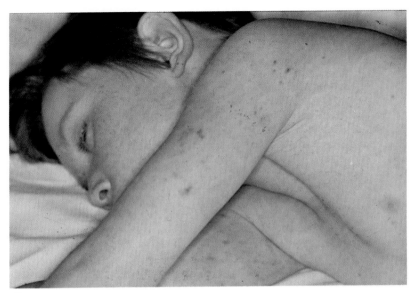

65

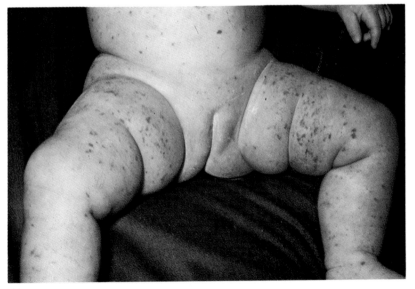

66

67   Meningitis – close-up of rash. On histological examination the capillaries and small arterioles in the skin lesions are dilated and engorged. The endothelial lining of the vessels is swollen, and many cells are packed with meningococci. Perivascular infiltration and haemorrhage complete the picture.

68   Fulminating infection. In about 10% of patients the septicaemia is overwhelming and there is little or no evidence of meningitis. Such a devastating attack manifests with high fever, shock and extensive purpura, especially over the face and extremities, and is usually accompanied by laboratory evidence of disseminated intravascular coagulation (DIC). Note the severe bleeding into the skin of this patient with DIC.

69   Disseminated intravascular coagulation. In fulminant cases DIC results in ischaemic damage to tissues, and extensive bleeding contributes to death; in less severe cases the clotting mechanisms are restored to normal as the infection responds to treatment. Diagnosis is established by measuring a number of parameters. Fragmented, burred, microspherocytic, and helmet-shaped erythrocytes are usually seen on freshly made blood films; platelets are reduced in number; prothrombin and thrombin times are prolonged; fibrin-degradation products are increased.

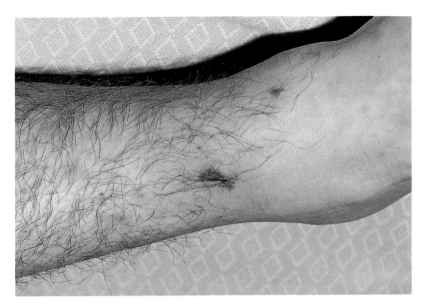

67

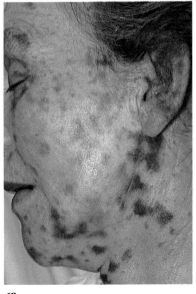

68

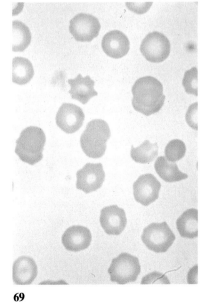

69

70 Chronic meningococcal septicaemia. The illness usually follows a prolonged benign course, characterised by recurrent bouts of fever accompanied by fleeting joint pains and crops of spots, but occasionally terminates in meningitis. The rash is seldom profuse and consists of discrete macules, papules, petechiae, and even small vesicles or pustules. Occasionally a rash on the legs resembling erythema nodosum is seen. A similar picture may be produced by chronic gonococcal septicaemia (see **184**), although in this condition haemorrhages are less prominent. The diagnosis is confirmed by blood culture, but several attempts may be necessary to recover the organism.

Complications

71 Waterhouse–Friderichsen syndrome – haemorrhage into suprarenal glands. Patients with fulminating meningococcal septicaemia may develop signs of peripheral circulatory failure, advancing rapidly to profound shock and death. When death is precipitate the rash may be scanty; when the patient survives longer there may be widespread bleeding.

At autopsy the common finding is gross haemorrhage into the suprarenal glands accompanied by thromboses of the large medullary veins. Frank haemorrhage may be absent in some patients dying from septicaemic shock, although degenerative changes may be present in the cortex; in others there may be no evidence of suprarenal damage. The suprarenal lesion may occasionally be only one of many caused by widespread DIC. The Waterhouse–Friderichsen syndrome is found in other severe infections.

In the illustration the suprarenal glands have been replaced by large clots of blood. (A = clots in suprarenal glands , B = kidneys.)

72 Meningitis – necrosis of skin (purpura necrotica). In severe infection thromboses in the intensely inflamed blood vessels of the skin may result in ischaemia, especially over pressure points. Profuse bleeding into the skin is followed by extensive necrosis, with sloughing of skin and subcutaneous tissues causing deep ulceration.

73 Meningitis – ulceration of skin. Healing is usually slow and skin grafting may be necessary. Keloid may form in the scar tissue.

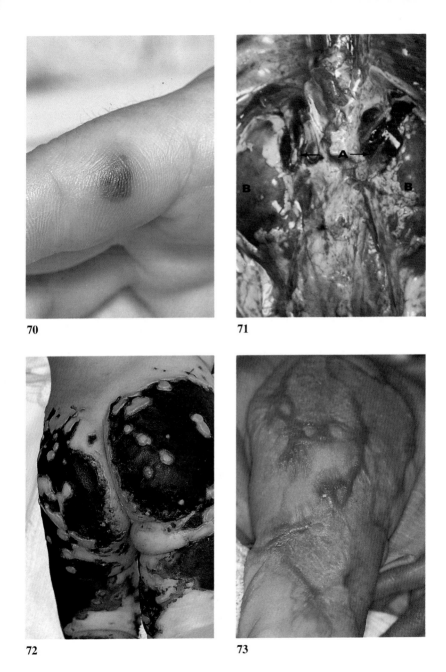

70

71

72

73

74   Squint following meningitis. Damage to cranial nerves can occur during the acute stage of the illness. The sixth cranial nerve, in its long course across the base of the brain, is particularly vulnerable, and paralysis of the external rectus muscle may be detected at an early stage. The weakness usually improves rapidly, and complete recovery takes place within a few weeks.

Extension of infection into the inner ear may cause partial or complete deafness.

75   Meningitis – iridochoroiditis. Serious damage to the eye is fortunately very rare with modern chemotherapy. Conjunctivitis, once common, resolves rapidly with treatment. Iridochoroiditis is more serious and may progress to panophthalmitis with risk of permanent blindness.

76   Meningitis – arthritis. The deposition of immune complexes at a late stage of the illness may result in pericarditis or arthritis with involvement of the large joints such as the knee. The effusion into the joint is viscous and contains a predominance of pus cells but the organism is seldom found. Fleeting joint pains are common in chronic meningococcal septicaemia.

The patient in the illustration developed arthritis in both knees on the fifth day of illness, while undergoing treatment for meningococcal meningitis. Although the effusion contained pus cells it proved to be sterile on culture.

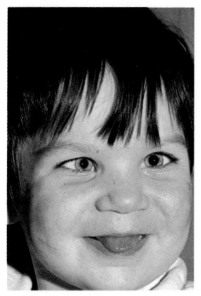

74

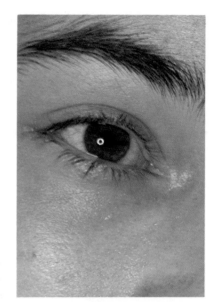

75

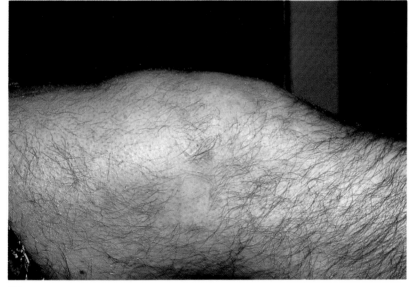

76

77   Pericarditis – chest radiograph. Endocarditis, myocarditis and pericarditis may be found during the course of acute meningococcal infection. Pericarditis is a rare complication and may be discovered unexpectedly at autopsy of patients dying from sudden overwhelming infection. Pericarditis, developing during the course of treatment, is associated with the deposition of immune complexes; the effusion is usually sterile.

This chest radiograph shows the typical globular shadow of a pericardial effusion that developed during the early convalescent stage of meningitis, while the patient was still under treatment. Treatment was continued and the pericarditis subsided uneventfully.

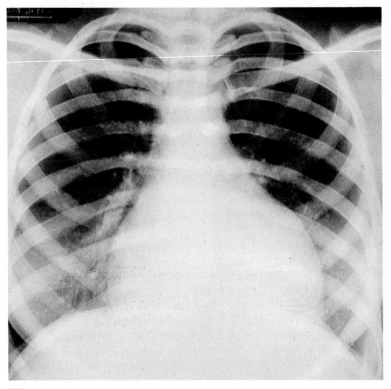

77

Pertussis (whooping cough)

Pertussis has long ranked among the most serious of the common infectious diseases of childhood. Permanent disability and even death may follow complications such as bronchopneumonia, lung collapse and encephalopathy. Apnoeic attacks in infants may cause brain damage and may end fatally.

Bordetella pertussis and *Bordetella parapertussis* are usually regarded as the causative organisms, although certain viruses, notably adenoviruses, parainfluenza, and respiratory syncytial virus have been associated with clinical states indistinguishable from pertussis. Pertussis is endemic and occurs throughout the year. Epidemics take place unpredictably every few years and may be related to the emergence of new or virulent strains of the organism. Although any age group may be affected, the disease predominantly involves young children. Mortality is highest in children under 1 year of age, especially when they are poorly nourished. Adults may also be infected, particularly in immunised communities.

Infection is spread by direct contact with oropharyngeal discharges, or by airborne droplets from the respiratory tract of children, particularly in the prodromal stage of the disease; school-aged children are frequently the source of infection for younger siblings at home. The organism enters the respiratory tract, where it adheres to the epithelium of the trachea and bronchi causing cell damage and interfering with ciliary action. Secretions and cell debris may block small air passages, causing lobular collapse and secondary infection. The organism does not invade the bloodstream.

The illness varies greatly in severity, and tends to run a protracted course. The initial catarrhal phase is accompanied by a simple cough, which alters in character as the illness progresses gradually into the paroxysmal stage. When fully developed the paroxysms consist of a series of coughs terminating in a characteristic 'whoop', frequently accompanied by vomiting. Bouts of paroxysms in rapid succession may leave the child exhausted, and repeated vomiting may lead to progressive weakness from malnutrition. The patient's temperature remains normal in an uncomplicated attack of pertussis. In most cases the paroxysmal stage gradually abates, although a residual cough with a whoop may persist for many months, and even after coughing has ceased paroxysms may recur if the child develops an intercurrent respiratory virus infection.

Organism

78 *Bordetella pertussis* **colonies on Lacey's modification of Bordet–Gengou medium. Incubation for 3 days at 37°C.** The usual shape of *Bordetella pertussis* is a short, thick, oval rod, but filamentous forms may be found in old cultures. The organism is Gram-negative and a strict aerobe. Enriched media are required for primary isolation. After 24 hours small transparent colonies may be detected. These grow larger on further incubation and become opaque and greyish. There are three serotypes.

Bordetella pertussis is recovered most readily from pernasal swabs taken during the first two weeks of illness. Cough plates give less successful results.

Clinical features

79 **Subconjunctival haemorrhage.** The subconjunctival collections of blood retain their bright red colour because oxygen diffuses easily across the thin membrane and saturates the haemoglobin. The blood is absorbed after a week or two, and no permanent harm results.

80 **Subconjunctival haemorrhages.** During a violent paroxysm of coughing the intrathoracic pressure rises sharply and affects the venous return to the heart. The sudden surge in capillary pressure may rupture the poorly supported subconjunctival vessels and cause an alarming haemorrhage. Secondary rise in intra-abdominal pressure may precipitate a hernia or rectal prolapse; both complications are rare. Children with severe pertussis frequently have a slightly cyanotic tinge due to inadequate oxygenation of the blood circulating through collapsed lung tissue.

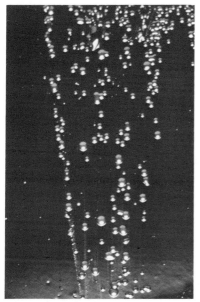

78

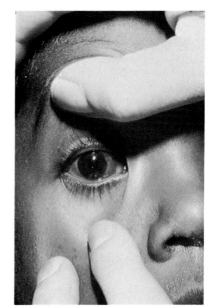

79

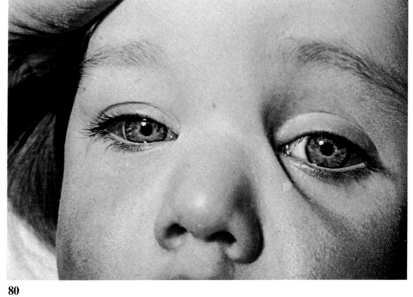

80

81 **Frenal ulcer.** During paroxysms of coughing in young children the tongue may be protruded against the sharp lower teeth, causing a small traumatic ulcer on the frenum.

82 **Chest radiograph, showing patchy collapse and consolidation (PA view).**

83 **Chest radiograph, showing collapse of left lower lobe.** *B. pertussis* occasionally causes a primary bronchopneumonia; more frequently it paves the way for secondary bacterial invasion from the upper respiratory tract. Plugs of sticky mucus may block the bronchi and bronchioles, causing lung collapse. Many patches of atelectasis are fleeting; others become infected by pyogenic bacteria and secondary pneumonia follows. The outlook has been improved by modern chemotherapy, and collapse is seldom permanent. In prospective studies there is little evidence that lung damage in pertussis commonly leads to bronchiectasis.

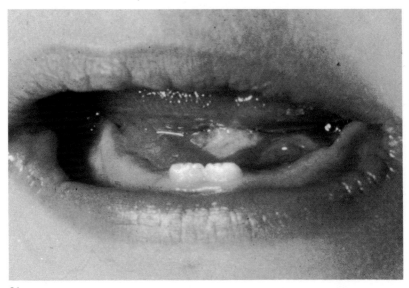

81

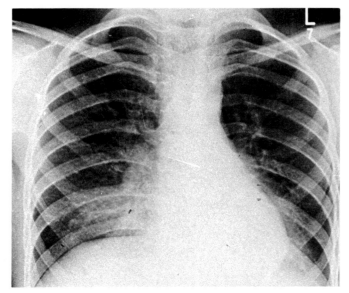

82

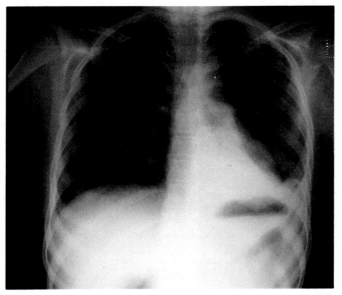

83

Salmonella infection

Salmonellae are intestinal parasites and have been detected in a great variety of hosts, including mammals, birds, amphibia, and reptiles. A few salmonellae are host-specific; most are not. In humans salmonellae are responsible for typhoid and paratyphoid fevers, and are the most common cause of bacterial food poisoning in North America and some European countries. Salmonella food poisoning is very common in countries with intensive rearing of food animals, mass production of food, and mass catering. Many cases of salmonella gastroenteritis are sporadic but food-borne outbreaks are common and are usually associated with restaurants, canteens, hospitals, and institutions. The source of infection is usually meat, poultry or eggs contaminated by the intestinal contents of infected livestock. Contamination of food by an infected person is unusual; direct person-to-person spread is common in hospitals and institutions. In most attacks the organism is confined to the bowel, where it causes acute vomiting and diarrhoea; in a few patients the salmonella may invade the bloodstream and result in metastatic infection of the meninges, bones, or joints.

Typhoid and paratyphoid fevers (enteric fever)

Typhoid fever is a generalised infection caused by *Salmonella typhi*; paratyphoid fever is caused by *Salmonella paratyphi* A, B, and C. All four are human parasites, though *S. paratyphi* B has been described in cattle. Both typhoid and paratyphoid infections are derived ultimately from the faeces or urine of a human case or carrier, and the organisms are usually transmitted by contaminated water or food.

Organism

84   Electron micrograph of a salmonella. Salmonellae are Gram-negative, non-sporing bacilli measuring 2–4 μm in length. They are actively motile and have numerous long peritrichate flagellae. Most strains are fimbriate, and capsules are rarely formed. Under the Kauffmann–White classification salmonellae may be categorised by identification of flagellar (H), somatic (O), and (in some freshly isolated strains, particularly of *S. typhi*), by virulence (Vi) antigens. Vi-positive strains of *S. typhi* can usually be phage typed and this technique has proved to be very useful epidemiologically.

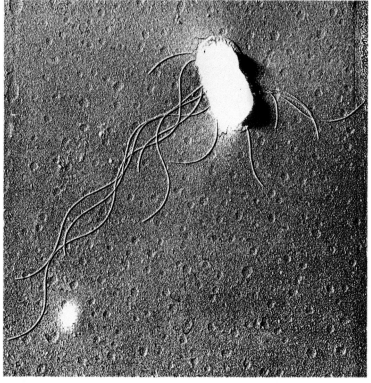

84

Clinical features of enteric fever

85 **'Step-ladder' temperature chart of typhoid fever.** The onset of the disease is generally insidious with lethargy, malaise, frontal headache, muscular aching, and joint pains. A dry cough is common and may lead to a misdiagnosis of bronchitis or pneumonia. The temperature rises in a step-ladder fashion, reaching its highest point at the end of a week. The pyrexia continues unabated throughout the second and third weeks. When the outcome is favourable the temperature falls slowly by lysis, returning to normal in the fourth week. During the first week the pulse rate is not increased in proportion to the rise in temperature and rarely exceeds 100/min.

86 **Distribution of rose-spot rash.** The typical rash of typhoid fever may appear towards the end of the first week but it has been recorded as late as the 20th day. It is present in about half the adults with typhoid but is less common in children.

The rash is distributed over the abdomen and chest and may extend to the back and proximal parts of the limbs but is rarely seen on the face, hands, or feet. The rash is not itchy. To assist identification, the rose spots on this patient have been ringed.

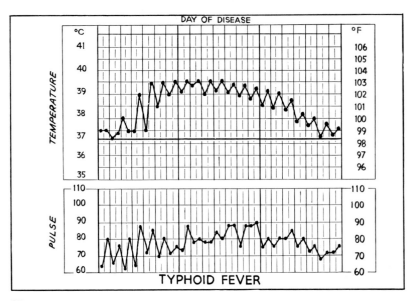

85

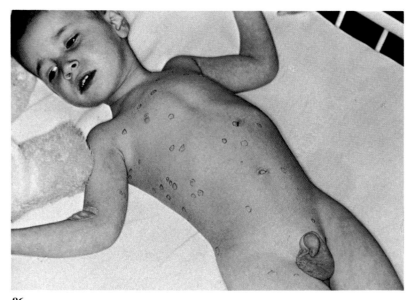

86

87   Rose spots in paratyphoid fever. The rose spots in paratyphoid fever tend to be larger than those found in typhoid, and the rash often has a maculopapular appearance. When the rash is heavy it may be mistaken for measles or infectious mononucleosis. Careful consideration of the history and other signs should prevent this error.

88   Rose spots on the abdomen in typhoid fever. The rash in typhoid fever consists of discrete pinkish macules or maculopapules, 2–4 mm in diameter. The lesions appear in crops over a period of 1–4 days, and individual lesions persist for 3 or 4 days. The spots tend to reappear during relapses and have even been observed during convalescence.

Rose spots are nearly impossible to detect on dark skins; when scanty they are easily overlooked on pale skins. Two rose spots on the side of this patient's abdomen have been ringed so that fresh lesions may be recognised when they emerge.

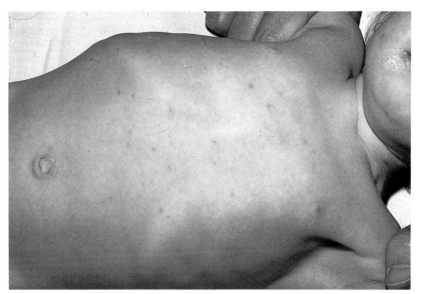

87

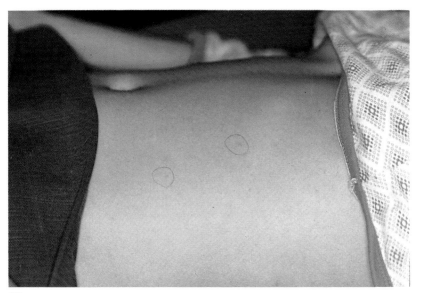

88

89   Close-up of rose spots. Rose spots consist of pinkish macules or maculopapules, measuring 2–4 mm in diameter. They blanch on pressure. A drop of oil on a rose spot increases the intensity of the colour and renders it more prominent.

90   Typhoid abdomen. During the first week of the illness most patients complain of some abdominal discomfort. As the attack progresses the abdomen becomes more distended, and is tender and tumid on palpation. The initial constipation gives way to diarrhoea in nearly one-third of patients.

The diagnosis of typhoid or paratyphoid fever is confirmed most reliably by blood culture; the organism may also be cultured from stool and occasionally from urine. Antibodies may be detected in the patient's serum against H and O antigens. This forms the basis of the Widal test for typhoid and paratyphoid fevers. The results of this serological test must be interpreted with caution, especially in areas where enteric fever is endemic and subclinical infection common.

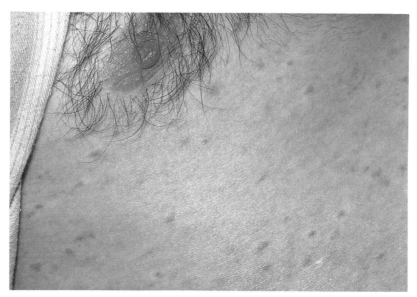

89

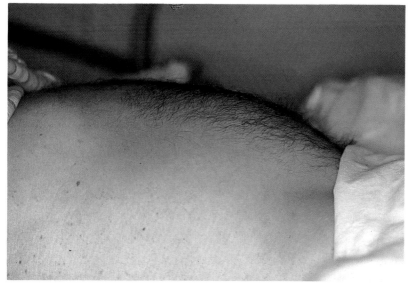

90

Complications of enteric fever and other salmonella infections

91 **Plain radiograph of the abdomen in paralytic ileus.** In the second or third week of typhoid fever the patient may develop paralytic ileus with increasing distension of the abdomen and persistent vomiting. A plain radiograph of the abdomen may show dilated loops of bowel with fluid levels. This complication usually responds to standard medical treatment with gastric suction and intravenous infusion to maintain water and electrolyte balance.

92 **Ulcerated Peyer's patches.** During the first week of typhoid fever the Peyer's patches in the small bowel become swollen and hyperaemic. The lymphoid tissue is infiltrated by large numbers of macrophages derived from the reticuloendothelial system. The intervening mucosa usually appears to be normal but may sometimes be acutely inflamed.

In severe attacks the lymphoid tissue undergoes necrosis, and a slough forms that separates during the third week to leave a characteristic ulcer. These ulcers are most numerous in the terminal ileum and lie in the long axis of the bowel. Most are confined to the mucosa or submucosa, but some penetrate the muscular and serous layers giving rise to haemorrhage and perforation. In favourable cases the ulcers heal by granulation, with minimal scarring.

93 **Histology of bowel in typhoid fever (haematoxylin and eosin stain).** Many large, rounded mononuclear cells are present. These modified histiocytes have abundant opaque cytoplasm and are sometimes referred to as 'typhoid cells'. In addition, there are moderate numbers of lymphocytes, but polymorphonuclear leucocytes are rare. (A = 'typhoid cell'; B = lymphocyte.)

94 **Plain radiograph of the gallbladder.** Chronic cholecystitis may follow an acute attack of typhoid fever, or may develop insidiously in later years. In either event it may perpetuate the carrier state, especially when associated with cholelithiasis. Cholecystectomy alone may clear the infection in 68–90% of chronic faecal carriers. Acute cholecystitis is found in under 2% of cases of typhoid fever and is more frequently seen in women, particularly obese or older women.

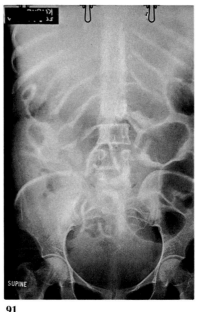

91

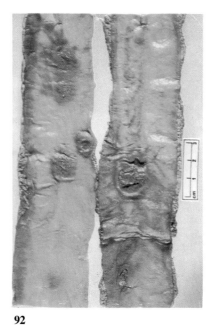

92

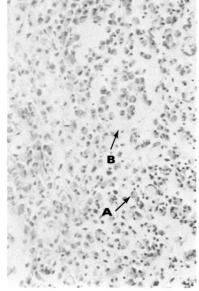

93

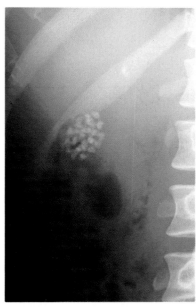

94

81

95 Chart – relapse and treatment. The rate of relapse in untreated typhoid fever varies from 5 to 15%. If the organism is sensitive to chloramphenicol and this antibiotic is given for less than 14 days the rate of relapse is greatly increased and may exceed 50%. Using a longer course of treatment fewer than 10% of patients relapse.

Relapses usually take place 7–10 days after the temperature has returned to normal but are often delayed in patients treated with antibiotics, and have even been recorded after 3 weeks of normal temperature. Relapses are generally milder and of shorter duration than the original attack but may be severe and prove fatal. The illness follows a pattern similar to the primary attack, and rose spots may reappear.

96 Typhoid spine. Radiograph of lumbar spine – AP view. Osteomyelitis and arthritis are rare complications of typhoid fever. Periostitis may by found in late convalescence, usually affecting the tibia or ribs. Abscesses may form and discharge pus containing the typhoid bacillus.

Osteomyelitis of the spine may follow an attack of typhoid fever. In some instances it is caused directly by the typhoid bacillus; in others by secondary infection with the tubercle bacillus. The radiograph shows involvement of L4 and L5 with deposition of new bone.

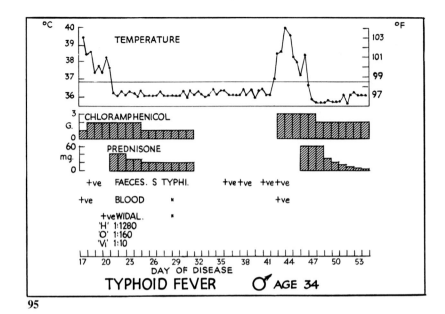

95

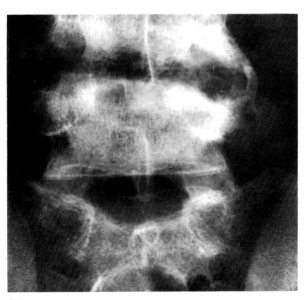

96

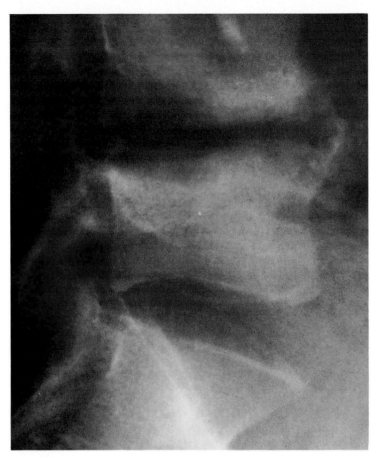

97

97   Typhoid spine. Radiograph of lumbar vertebra – lateral view.
This view of the spine shows areas of decalcification and irregular
deposition of new bone in the fifth lumbar vertebra of a patient with a
typhoid infection.

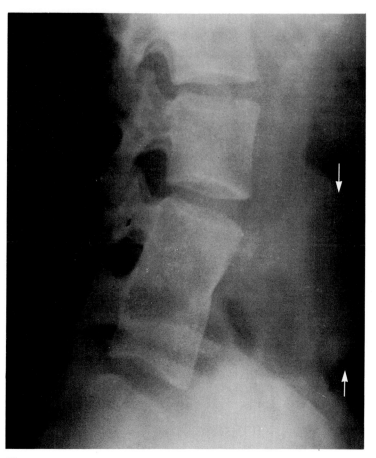

98

98 Osteomyelitis of spine and psoas abscess in paratyphoid B.
Infection with paratyphoid B is more likely to cause a suppurative
lesion, such as osteomyelitis, than paratyphoid A. The lateral view of the
lumbar spine shows a large psoas abscess, which originated from a
paratyphoid infection of L4 and L5. The vertebral bodies are fused.
Although the attack of paratyphoid occurred many years previously, the
organism was cultured from the pus drained at operation. (The arrows
indicate the abscess.)

99   Sickle-cell anaemia with paratyphoid osteomyelitis. Patients with sickle-cell disease are especially prone to salmonella infections of bone. Salmonella osteomyelitis usually occurs in children. It commonly affects long bones and may affect more than one.

The radiograph shows characteristic changes of osteomyelitis in a young child with paratyphoid B infection of the radius and ulna. Note the patchy decalcification and the periosteal reaction.

100   Sickle-cell disease with osteomyelitis complicating food poisoning. Radiograph of tibia. Osteomyelitis may complicate salmonella food poisoning in patients with sickle-cell disease. The diagnosis is not easy, but the possibility should always be considered if a patient with sickle-cell anaemia has persistent fever and localised pain during or after an attack of salmonella food poisoning. Blood cultures may confirm systemic invasion by a salmonella, but 3 weeks or more may elapse before radiographic changes can be detected. However, bone scans may confirm the diagnosis at an earlier stage.

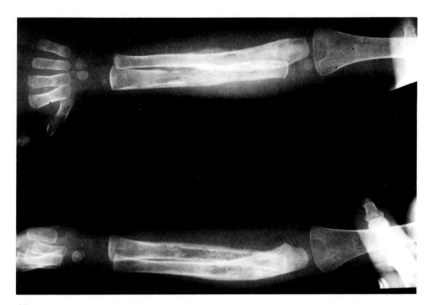

99

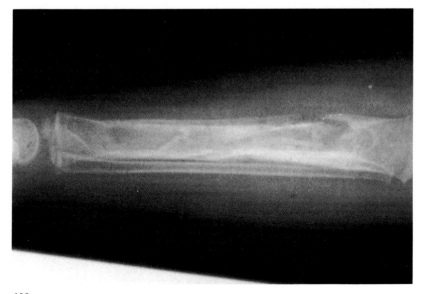

100

Gastroenteritis

Gastroenteritis varies greatly according to the aetiology of the infection and the age of the patient. In infants and young children vomiting and diarrhoea rapidly lead to dehydration with imbalance of electrolytes, consequently gastroenteritis is a serious disease with an appreciable mortality rate. In older children and adults the disease may be incapacitating but is seldom fatal. The clinical features of many types of gastroenteritis are very similar and it is difficult on clinical assessment to be certain of the nature of the infection.

Enteropathogenic strains of *Escherichia coli* (EPEC) cause infantile gastroenteritis and enterotoxic strains (ETEC) are associated with traveller's diarrhoea in all ages. Campylobacters, vibrio-like microaerophilic Gram-negative bacteria, are another very common cause of gastroenteritis affecting all age groups, and are probably an important cause of traveller's diarrhoea. Several small viruses not yet grown on tissue culture are important causes of diarrhoea, especially in young children. These viruses include rotavirus (wheel-like), astrovirus (five- or six-pointed star), calicivirus (calyx), parvovirus (small round viruses) and viruses commonly associated with respiratory tract infections such as adenovirus and coronaviruses.

101 Electron micrograph of rotaviruses. Rotavirus gastroenteritis is a common condition worldwide. It usually affects infants and young children but may involve all age groups. Fever and vomiting may be present for up to 48 hours before the onset of diarrhoea, which is very variable and may be minimal in older children. Respiratory symptoms are present in 40% of cases. A double-stranded RNA virus with a characteristic wheel-like appearance may be detected by electron microscopy of faeces during the acute stage. During convalescence, antibody is demonstrated by the ability of serum to agglutinate faecal virus particles (immune electron microscopy).

Clinical features

102 Dehydration – mild. In mild dehydration there may be loss of up to 5% of body weight. The baby is irritable and cries miserably. As a result of vasoconstriction the skin is pale, but the lips remain a vivid pink because of haemoconcentration.

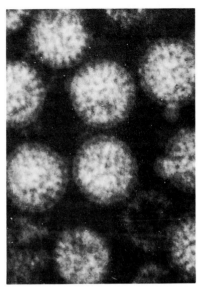

101

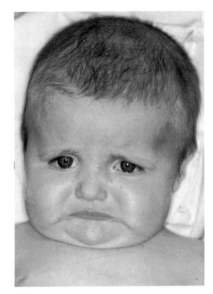

102

103 Dehydration – moderate. In moderate dehydration up to 10% of the body weight may be lost. Pallor is still a striking feature, but irritability gives way to listlessness as dehydration increases. Water is lost from the retro-orbital pad of fat, and the eyes become sunken. The fontanelle is depressed, and the mouth parched.

104 Dehydration – moderate. The skin loses its turgor and elasticity. Normally when a fold of skin is pinched and then released, it subsides immediately but in dehydration it settles very slowly. This phenomenon can be seen clearly on the anterior abdominal wall of this child. Note the wrinkled skin.

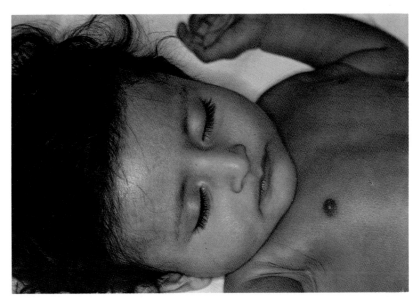

103

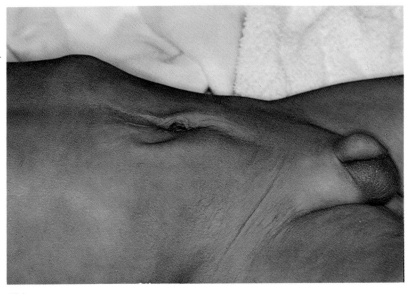

104

105 and 106   Dehydration – severe. In extreme dehydration, when 10–15% of the body weight has been lost, peripheral circulatory failure supervenes. The child is limp and apathetic. The extremities feel icy cold, and the peripheral pulses are absent. Drowsiness gives way to coma. Finally, the child lies as if dead with eyeballs rolled upwards, and sclerae showing white between the half-closed eyelids. Oliguria is invariably present, and the blood urea concentration rises rapidly. Bleeding may occur into the gastrointestinal tract. Acidosis is usually present. The mortality in such severely dehydrated patients is 50%.

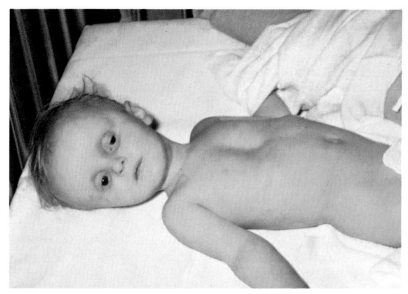

105

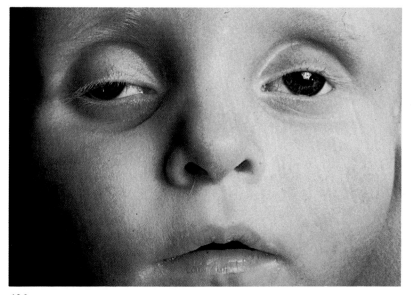

106

107 Hypernatraemia – conjunctival congestion. Hypernatraemic dehydration may be suspected clinically when a dehydrated child is exceptionally irritable or has a neck stiffness. Convulsions are common in this group, especially when the dehydration is corrected rapidly with hypotonic infusions. Permanent brain damage or death may result. Conjunctival congestion is a common finding in these patients. The diagnosis should be confirmed by measuring the serum electrolyte concentrations.

108 Marasmus following an attack of gastroenteritis. In severe gastroenteritis the infant may become intolerant to all types of oral feeding and enter a chronic state of dehydration and wasting from malnutrition. Despite intravenous feeding mortality remains high, varying from 10 to 50% in different outbreaks. Temporary lactose intolerance is not uncommon after severe gastroenteritis. In such patients the reintroduction of milk into the diet exacerbates diarrhoea.

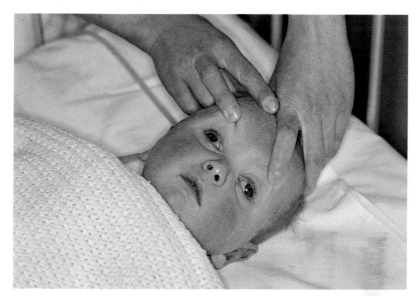

107

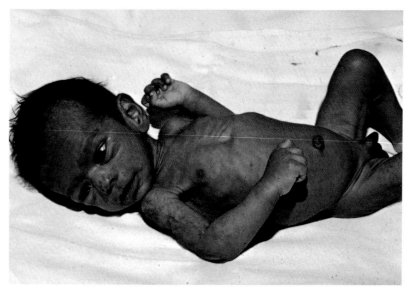

108

Diphtheria

Corynebacterium diphtheriae, the causative organism of diphtheria, grows on the surface of the body and produces a powerful polypeptide exotoxin that is absorbed and carried in the circulation to the heart and nervous system, where it causes cellular damage by interfering with protein synthesis. Human cases or carriers are the sole source of infection, which is spread by close contact, the organism being transferred by infected secretions or very occasionally by fomites. Infection is worldwide, mainly in children, but is rare in countries with effective childhood immunisation programmes.

Organism

109 *Corynebacterium diphtheriae mitis* **(Albert's stain of smear).** *C. diphtheriae* is a slender, non-motile, non-sporing, Gram-positive bacillus, measuring 3–5 μm in length. It can be classified into three types, mitis, intermedius, and gravis, according to (a) the appearance of the colonies on blood-tellurite media, (b) biochemical reactions, and (c) staining characteristics.

The staining reaction by Albert's method is uneven, and metachromatic granules are often present. These may be bipolar or scattered irregularly throughout the protoplasm; pleomorphism is common. In contrast, diphtheroid bacilli are much more regular in appearance. The morphological appearances, however, cannot be relied upon to distinguish one type of diphtheria bacillus from another, or diphtheria bacilli from diphtheroids. Cultural and biochemical characteristics must be taken into account.

110 *Corynebacterium diphtheriae gravis*. **Smear from culture.** The arrangement of diphtheria bacilli is distinctive. They may be found singly or in groups. In groups the organisms tend to be arranged at angles to each other, probably as a result of incomplete separation at the moment of division. They look like the letters L or V, and the combinations bear a resemblance to Chinese or cuneiform writing.

109

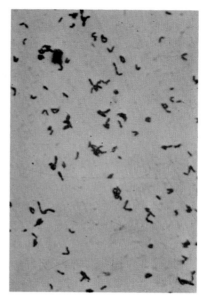

110

111   Colonies of *C. diphtheriae* on McLeod's medium (× 4.4). On McLeod's chocolate tellurite agar the three types (mitis, intermedius, and gravis) produce characteristic colonies. Mitis are black, shiny, and dome-shaped; intermedius has pointed, pinhead-sized colonies; gravis has dull matt colonies with a central dome and a crenated edge resembling a daisy head. All strains ferment glucose but not sucrose; gravis alone ferments starch. However, it should be noted that differentiation into mitis, intermedius and gravis strains is not a reliable guide to toxigenicity.

The diphtheria bacillus may be divided serologically into many subtypes and classified by bacteriophage into at least 19 types. Some strains of mitis are avirulent but may produce exotoxin under the influence of bacteriophages.

112   Elek plate. Toxigenic strains may be identified by immunodiffusion. A strip of filter paper, impregnated with antitoxin, is set in culture medium and diphtheria bacilli streaked on the surface at right angles to the paper. Toxin from the growing organisms diffuses sideways from the streaks, while antitoxin diffuses from the filter paper. A thin white line of precipitate marks the interface where antitoxin combines with toxin. This method is not as reliable as *in vivo* testing for virulence.

In the Elek plate illustrated the outer two organisms are non-toxigenic, the inner two are known to be toxigenic strains, and the central organism is being tested against these controls. A reaction can be seen between the lines produced by the suspect strain and the two control strains. There is no reaction from the outer non-toxigenic organisms.

113   Virulence test in the rabbit. Rabbits and guinea-pigs are highly susceptible to diphtheria toxin and may be used to test strains for virulence. The minimal lethal dose is determined by injecting various dilutions of toxin subcutaneously, and the minimal reacting dose is established by intradermal inoculation. Gravis and intermedius strains are nearly always virulent, whereas mitis strains are frequently avirulent.

A few positive reactions are present on the rabbit's skin 2 days after inoculation, but most are negative.

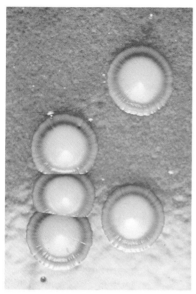

111

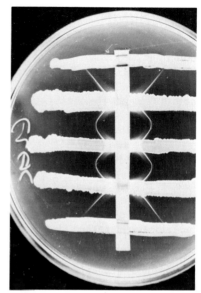

112

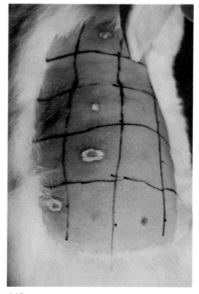

113

Clinical features

C. diphtheriae, growing on the surface of the body, causes local cellular damage resulting in the formation of a pseudomembrane. Toxin from the surface infection is absorbed into the bloodstream and carried to the heart and nervous system, where it damages the cells and causes serious, though temporary, impairment of function. The clinical manifestations of diphtheria vary with the extent and site of the local lesion and the degree of damage to the heart and nervous system by exotoxin.

114 Nasal diphtheria. The possibility of diphtheria or a foreign body should always be considered when a child has a unilateral blood-stained discharge from the nose. In anterior nasal diphtheria the skin round the nostril or on the upper lip may be excoriated and membrane or crusting visible inside the nose.

Absorption of toxin is slight so there is no threat to life, but large numbers of diphtheria bacilli are shed and these patients are dangerous to others.

115 'Bull-neck' of diphtheria. Extensive diphtheria of the throat is always accompanied by marked swelling of the neck resulting from enlargement of lymph nodes and oedema of surrounding tissues. The swelling feels solid, and it is difficult to palpate the underlying lymph nodes. There is little pain.

116 Distinguishing between mumps and 'bull-neck' diphtheria. Failure to examine the throat of a child with 'bull-neck' diphtheria may lead to a mistaken and tragic diagnosis of mumps. The child with serious diphtheria looks pale, limp, and toxic, whereas the child with mumps looks comparatively well. Moreover, the swelling of mumps lies superior to that of diphtheria and usually fills the hollow behind the angle of the jaw. Careful inspection of the throat settles the diagnosis.

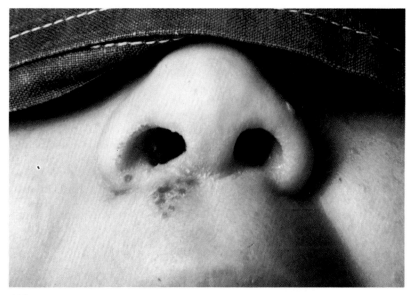

114

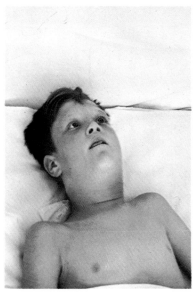

115

116

117　Tonsillar diphtheria. Membrane is confined to the tonsils, where absorption of toxin is moderate. It starts as a small patch on one tonsil and usually spreads to both. The membrane is ivory white or greyish yellow in colour. The edge is wrinkled but sharply demarcated, and bordered by a narrow band of inflammation. The child is listless and off-colour but may not complain of a sore throat, and the cause of the illness may be overlooked. Pyrexia is slight or absent.

118　Severe pharyngeal diphtheria. In severe diphtheria the membrane may be thin and transparent, especially at the spreading edge. The older parts of the membrane are usually greyish yellow, but if there has been bleeding into the membrane the colour may alter to green or black. The membrane is firmly adherent and forcible removal causes slight bleeding. The underlying mucosa is not ulcerated and membrane forms again after 24 hours. The fauces are oedematous.

119　Spread of membrane in pharyngeal diphtheria. Membrane spreads rapidly from the tonsils across the soft palate to the uvula and over the pharyngeal wall into the nasopharynx. Toxin is readily absorbed, and general symptoms are severe with waxy pallor, extreme lassitude, and drowsiness progressing to stupor. The patient's temperature may be subnormal, and death quickly ensues from circulatory failure.

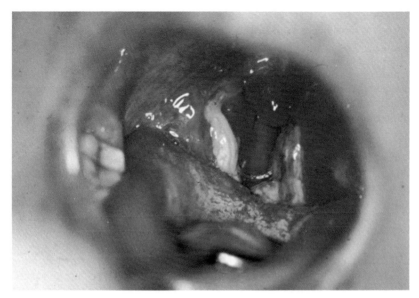

117

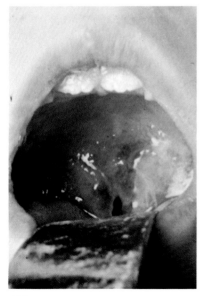

118

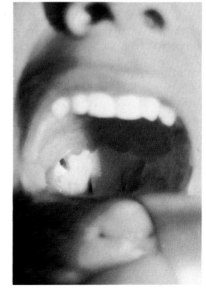

119

120 Anginose variety of infectious mononucleosis. The anginose form of infectious mononucleosis is of similar appearance to diphtheria, but the exudate usually retains a striking white hue and does not spread further than the tonsils. Despite the alarming exudate on the tonsils, the patient's general condition remains good. Generalised enlargement of lymph nodes and splenomegaly indicate the correct clinical diagnosis, which is confirmed by finding characteristic mononuclear cells in the blood and a positive Paul–Bunnell test or one of its simplified variants.

121 Laryngeal diphtheria. Diphtheria of the larynx may be primary or secondary to pharyngeal diphtheria. Toxic absorption is slight, and the illness is dominated by respiratory obstruction caused by the membrane. As breathing becomes more difficult the accessory muscles are brought into play, and the soft parts of the chest wall and supraclavicular fossae are sucked inwards. The child becomes restless and frightened as he struggles for breath. Eventually the violent muscular effort can no longer be sustained, the child falls back exhausted, and death swiftly follows.

Diagnosis of laryngeal diphtheria is easy when membrane is visible in the pharynx but otherwise presents difficulty. Viral forms of laryngitis are associated with catarrhal signs in other parts of the respiratory tract and generally have a more abrupt onset than diphtheria.

122 Histological appearances in diphtheritic tracheobronchitis. Diphtheria bacilli, multiplying on the respiratory mucosa, provoke an inflammatory response. The superficial tissues become infiltrated by leucocytes and fibrin-rich fluid exudes from the engorged vessels. The epithelial cells die and are enmeshed with the bacteria in a coagulum of protein to form a membrane. In the lower respiratory tract, where the ciliated epithelium is loosely attached, the membrane is easily dislodged and may be coughed out at tracheotomy or impacted in the larynx. (A = membrane; B = submucosa infiltrated by leucocytes; C = cartilage ring.)

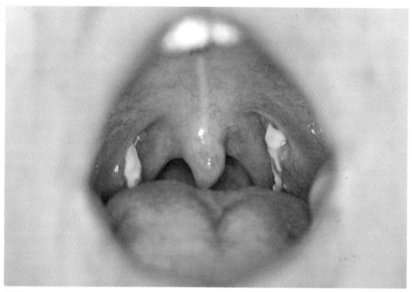

120

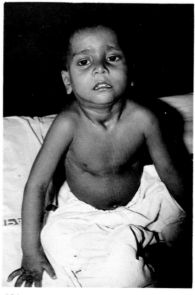

121

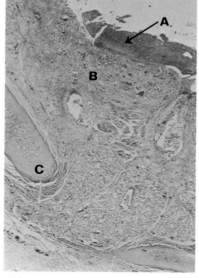

122

Complications

Diphtheritic neuropathy is caused by toxic damage to motor nerves and appears sequentially. Palatal paresis develops about days 14–21; ocular paresis before day 28; paralysis of muscles of larynx, pharynx or respiration between days 36 and 42; paralysis of limbs as late as day 70. Ultimate recovery is assured.

123 Histology of the heart in diphtheria. Diphtheria toxin, by interfering with protein synthesis, damages cardiac muscle cells with resultant fatty degeneration. The patchy areas of damaged myocardium soon become surrounded and infiltrated by leucocytes, many of which are macrophages. In surviving patients fibroblastic repair results in microscopic scars but these do not seem to impair cardiac function.

124 Electrocardiographic changes in diphtheria. Toxic damage to the heart manifests clinically about the eighth to tenth day but may appear earlier in severe cases. The first signs are tachycardia and an irregular pulse. Inverted T waves or alterations in the ST segment are to be expected in the early stage, and complete heart block may ensue. Restlessness, pallor, vomiting, precordial pain and oliguria are grave prognostic signs. Death commonly occurs about the fifteenth day; survival beyond this stage makes the outlook more hopeful.

This electrocardiogram shows severe changes in a fatal case of diphtheria caused by a mitis strain. Nodal bradycardia is present with ventricular ectopic escape, depression of the ST segment, and inversion of T waves.

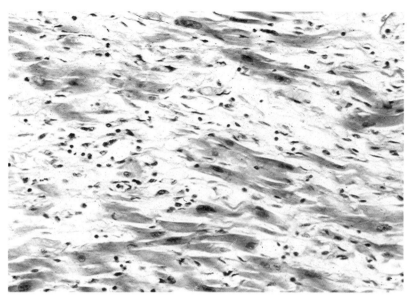

123

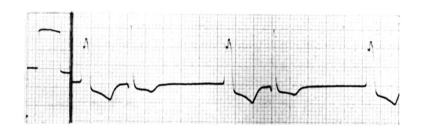

124

Vincent's infection

125 Vincent's organisms – dilute carbol fuchsin smear. A spirochaete and fusiform bacillus are found in large numbers in certain mouth lesions and in ulcerative or necrotic lesions elsewhere. The spirochaete, *Borrelia vincentii*, measures 7–18 μm in length and has 3–8 loose, open coils. It is actively motile and is an obligate anaerobe. The associated bacillus, *Fusibacterium fusiforme*, is cigar-shaped and measures 5–14 μm. It is non-motile and a strict anaerobe. Both organisms are easily detected in smears, stained by dilute carbol fuchsin, but are difficult to culture.

126 Vincent's angina. Vincent's organisms may be found in small numbers on healthy gums. They do not usually act as primary pathogens but as secondary invaders when superficial tissues have been damaged or are defective as a result of trauma, other infections, malnutrition, agranulocytosis or leukaemia. In temperate climates infection is confined to the buccal cavity or respiratory tract, but in tropical climates the organisms may be found in skin ulcers (see **394**).

In Vincent's angina membranous ulcers may be present on the tonsils or pharynx. Halitosis is a feature, but general disturbance is slight. Infection may spread to adjacent areas of the palate.

127 Acute ulcerative gingivitis. When the gums are involved there is destruction of the interdental papillae, leaving shallow concave ulcers with white necrotic margins. Vincent's infection may cause widespread destruction with extensive ulceration. The regional lymph nodes are enlarged.

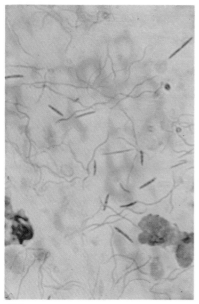

125

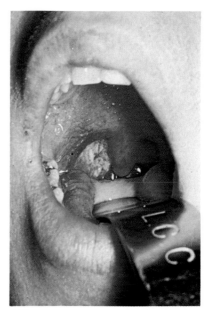

126

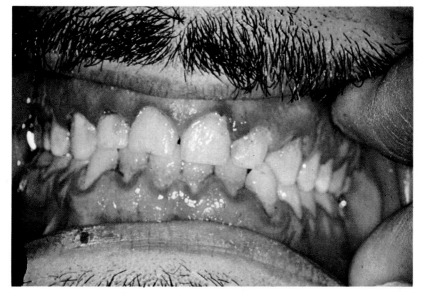

127

Thrush

128 *Candida albicans* – **Gram stain of smear from mouth.** *C. albicans* is a yeast-like fungus. In favourable conditions the fungus appears as spherical or oval yeast cells, called blastospores, which reproduce by budding; when conditions are less favourable it grows as a pseudomycelium of non-branching filamentous cells, which divide by constriction. Further yeast cells are formed by budding at the division sites; both forms are thin-walled. Some yeast cells become larger, develop thick walls, and enter a resting phase. These resting cells are termed chlamydospores. *C. albicans* is a Gram-positive organism.

129 *Candida albicans* – **Gram stain of smear showing yeast cells from 48 hour growth on blood agar at 37°C.** *Candida albicans* is found in humans, animals and birds. It is a common surface commensal in humans and is present in the mouth and faeces of 20–30% of healthy people. Superficial infection of skin or mucous membranes occurs in debilitated patients or when there has been local disturbance as a result of infection or antibiotic treatment. Deep-seated infections and chronic superficial infections may complicate disorders of immunity.

130 Oral thrush. Thrush of the mouth may be found in infants as a result of cross-infection from the mother or from other infants, particularly in bottle-fed babies. Environmental contamination is especially common in nurseries. In adults, infection is usually endogenous and is found in dehydrated or debilitated patients, or when the bacterial flora of the buccal cavity has been disturbed by antibiotic therapy. The raw inflamed mucous membrane is covered with patches of creamy-white exudate.

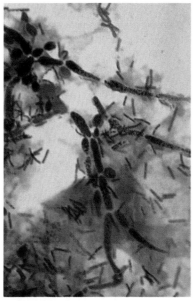

128

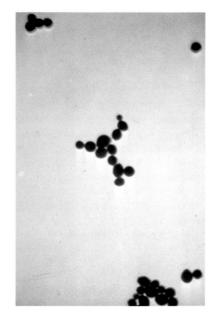

129

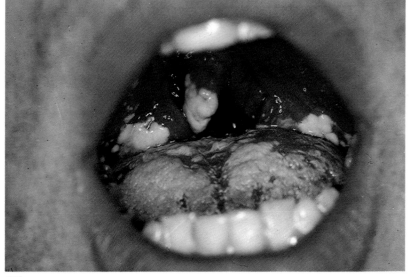

130

131 Chronic oral thrush. Chronic infection of the mouth may be associated with immunodeficiency. Firm diffuse white plaques, or numerous white papules with intervening erythema may be found in the buccal cavity. These may persist for months or years, depending on the nature of the underlying deficiency (see **336**).

132 Vulvovaginitis. Nappy rash in babies may be caused by candida and is particularly common in those with diarrhoea or those receiving antibiotic treatment. The rash starts round the anus and spreads over the perineum affecting skin in contact with the nappy. There is a well defined area of redness with raised edges. Satellite lesions may begin as small pustules that rupture to leave small raw patches. The skin is macerated. In an ammoniacal rash the skin folds tend to be spared.

Genital thrush may prove troublesome in women using oral contraceptives or during pregnancy. Redness of the vagina and labia may be accompanied by severe pruritus and scanty or thick white discharge.

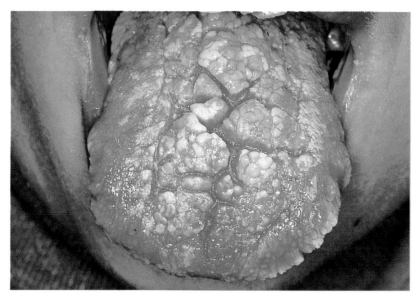

131

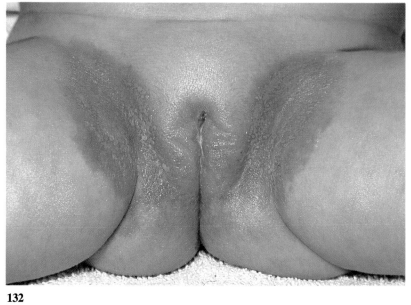

132

133   Balanitis. Poor hygiene may result in severe irritation of the foreskin and glans with blistering and patches of thrush.

134   Paronychia. Candida infection may spread from the nail fold under the adjacent nails, causing deformity and even loss of the nail. It is especially common in those whose hands are frequently immersed in water, and in patients with diabetes or endocrine disorders. Nail infection as a manifestation of chronic mucocutaneous candidiasis may occur in patients with immunological defects. In this child the infection was caused by persistent thumb-sucking.

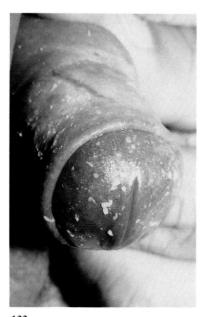

133

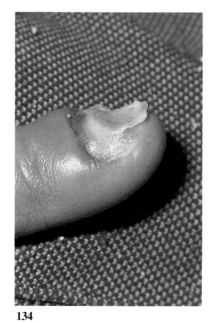

134

Mycobacterial infections

Tuberculosis

Tuberculosis is a disease of antiquity with a worldwide distribution, affecting not only humans but also many species of wild and domesticated animals. Tubercle bacilli are members of the genus *Mycobacterium*. Two species are chiefly responsible for tuberculosis in humans – the human strain, *Mycobacterium tuberculosis*, and the bovine strain, *Mycobacterium bovis*. Other mycobacteria, originally described as atypical, have also been found to be human pathogens, though generally of low virulence. The source of human tuberculosis is either an overt or subclinical case with bacteriologically positive sputum, or infected cattle. Infection is usually spread by airborne droplets, or by consumption of contaminated milk or its products. Respiratory disease due to *M. tuberculosis* is universal, but non-respiratory disease due to *M. bovis* is rare in countries with tuberculosis-free cattle herds and pasteurisation of milk. There has been an upsurge in infection with both *M. tuberculosis* and atypical mycobacteria in areas where HIV infection is prevalent.

135 Smear of sputum (Ziehl-Neelsen stain). Tubercle bacilli are slender rods, measuring 1–4 μm in length, which are stained with difficulty but once stained resist decolorisation by strong acids or alcohol. It is reasonable to make a presumptive diagnosis of tuberculosis if acid-fast bacilli are seen in sputum from a patient with radiological or clinical evidence of pulmonary disease, but it should be appreciated that acid-fast bacilli detected in clinical material are not necessarily tubercle bacilli, and also that negative microscopy does not exclude the diagnosis.

136 Smear of sputum (auramine-phenol stain). The Ziehl-Neelsen method is the classic technique for staining mycobacteria but other methods, such as auramine-phenol, have similar sensitivity and permit easier identification of mycobacteria.

137 Growth of tubercle bacilli. Mycobacteria require special media, such as Lowenstein–Jensen or pyruvate egg, and grow slowly to produce a friable tenacious mass of adherent organisms. Positive cultures are unlikely before 3 weeks and cultures should be maintained for at least 8 weeks. Identification depends on biochemical reactions, pigmentation, growth rate, and optimal growth temperature. Sputum for culture should be obtained after early morning deep cough. If sputum is not available, early morning gastric aspirates or secretions obtained at bronchoscopy are alternatives.

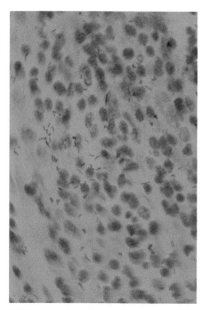

135

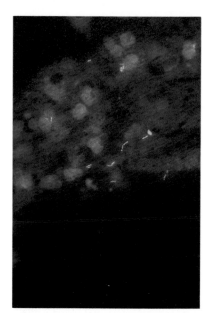

136

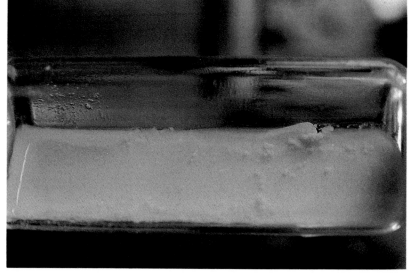

137

138 Mantoux reaction. Initial infection with the tubercle bacillus initiates a cell-mediated immune response to the tuberculoprotein of the bacillus. About 6 weeks after primary infection, challenge with an intradermal injection of tuberculin results in a delayed hypersensitivity skin reaction (type IV). The tuberculin skin test, such as the Mantoux or Heaf test, is an important and convenient method of identifying persons who have been infected with tubercle bacilli, although it does not identify those with active disease.

A strongly positive reaction is common in patients with recent infection, in non-pulmonary tuberculosis, and in those who are in continual contact with open tuberculosis. The reaction many be suppressed in Mantoux-positive individuals as a result of anergy caused by intercurrent infection, such as measles or infectious mononucleosis. The reaction may also be negative in patients with overwhelming tuberculosis or sarcoidosis, patients being treated with corticosteroids, and patients with deficient immunity, even when active tuberculosis is present.

139 Histology of tubercle. A tubercle is a typical allergic granuloma formed in response to non-soluble or poorly soluble antigens. At the centre of the lesion there is a Langhans-type of multinucleated giant cell, formed from macrophages induced to fuse together by lymphokines. The giant cell may contain tubercle bacilli and is surrounded by a zone of epithelioid cells, which are also derived from macrophages, and an outer shell of lymphocytes, macrophages, and plasma cells. Central necrosis follows and the remnants of dead cells have a caseous or cheese-like consistency. The growth of tubercle bacilli is greatly inhibited in the area of caseation. It is possible that hypoxia is one of the contributory factors because bacilli are more numerous towards the periphery. With effective treatment the lesions regress and are replaced by scar tissue. Calcium deposits are commonly laid down in caseous material.

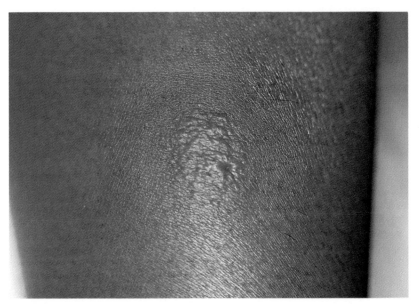

138

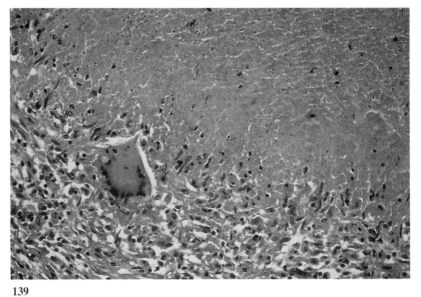

139

140 Primary complex – chest radiograph. In primary infection the inhaled tubercle bacilli usually lodge near the periphery of the lung, where they multiply and create a small area of inflammation, which slowly extends but remains unencapsulated (the Ghon focus). Bacilli may be carried to the regional lymph nodes. The combination of the local reaction and the enlarged regional lymph nodes is termed the primary complex. With the onset of cell-mediated hypersensitivity, the primary complex enlarges rapidly and may become caseous and walled off. When the outcome is favourable, the caseous material becomes inspissated and may calcify or disappear. Rarely in young children the lung component of the primary complex continues to increase in size and the caseous centre liquefies. The fluid contents may discharge into a bronchus, causing an acute diffuse tuberculous bronchopneumonia in one or both lungs, which frequently proves fatal. The nodal component shows less tendency to heal completely, and even after partial calcification living tubercle bacilli may persist for many years. In infants, particularly, infection may spread beyond the regional lymph nodes causing caseation in more distant nodes and eventual massive involvement of the mediastinal nodes. Infected nodes may become attached to a bronchus, leading to perforation of the bronchial wall and a fistula, or may compress and involve other structures. If a blood vessel is involved the wall is replaced by tuberculous granulation tissue and ulceration of the intimal lining may allow tubercle bacilli to escape into the bloodstream.

In infants and young children primary infection is commonly symptomless and may be detected only on routine radiological examination, or on tuberculin testing of contacts of known tuberculous patients. Any symptoms are likely to be of a general nature with malaise, anorexia, and loss of weight. In older children pyrexia and a cough may be present. The glandular component of the primary complex predominates, and consequently the air passages are likely to be compressed by enlarged lymph nodes, or occluded by endobronchitis or viscid sputum. The lung component may not be visible on radiographic examination of a young child and only the enlarged hilar glands may be seen. Obstruction of a bronchus may result in segmental, lobular or even complete collapse of a lung. In adults the lung component of the primary complex predominates. Sensitisation reactions, such as erythema nodosum or phlyctenular conjunctivitis, may draw attention to the underlying disease.

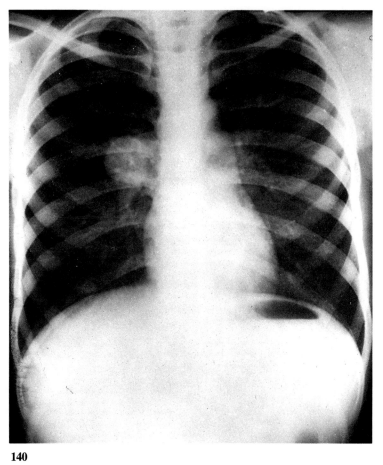

140

141 Miliary tuberculosis – chest radiograph. In both infants and adults with primary infection rapid invasion of the bloodstream may result in generalised miliary tuberculosis or tuberculous meningitis. Tubercle bacilli may be discharged into the bloodstream from a primary focus, or from a caseous gland rupturing into a pulmonary vein, artery or thoracic duct. The subsequent pathological reaction varies greatly: at one extreme there may be necrotic foci with little or no cellular reaction but containing many organisms; at the other a miliary tuberculosis with well developed tubercles containing few organisms. Once the primary lesion has healed and the gland focus calcified such spread is less likely. In the immunodeficient, massive dissemination of bacilli may take place, causing rapidly progressive disease which frequently is fatal.

Miliary tuberculosis usually follows within 6 months of primary infection. The onset is insidious with symptoms of general malaise, anorexia, loss of weight, irregular pyrexia, and a rising respiratory rate. Irritability and headache in a child or young adult, who remains unwell following the primary infection, should always arouse suspicion of miliary spread. On radiographic examination both lungs may be evenly and symmetrically involved with numerous circular foci measuring less than 5 mm in diameter. Choroid tubercles may be detected on ophthalmoscopy in about 25% of patients, and are a useful diagnostic sign. In a few patients with miliary tuberculosis the chest radiograph may be negative and choroid tubercles may not be detected. However, liver or bone-marrow biopsy may reveal tubercles and confirm the diagnosis. If investigations fail to yield positive results and the patient's condition continues to deteriorate, a therapeutic trial with anti-tuberculous drugs is justified, but before undertaking treatment gastric washings should be cultured for tubercle bacilli, even though the results cannot be available for some weeks.

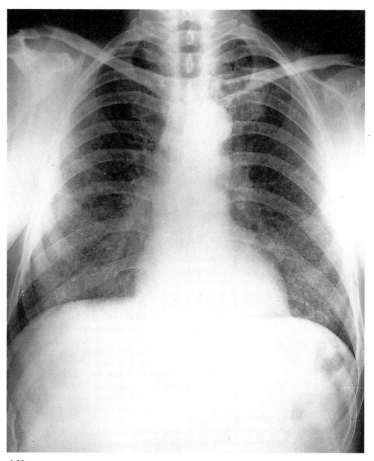

141

142 Choroid tubercles. Choroid tubercles may be the only immediately visible diagnostic sign of generalised miliary tuberculosis or tuberculous meningitis. One or more choroid tubercles may be seen on ophthalmoscopy. These are round or oval pale yellowish patches, about half the size of the optic disc, with an ill-defined border, and no visible retinal vessels passing over them.

143 Tuberculous lymphadenitis. Lymph nodes are frequently involved in primary infection and progressive enlargement may become the dominant feature of the primary complex. When the portal of entry is in the lung, the hilar glands may be involved; when the primary site is in the tonsils, the cervical lymph nodes may be enlarged; when the organism is ingested, the mesenteric nodes may be affected.

Tuberculous lymphadenitis is a common disease in some racial groups and may give rise to massive enlargement of mediastinal glands, or generalised lymphadenopathy and hepatosplenomegaly. Prolonged and recurrent fever may be the presenting features. In elderly persons enlargement of cervical lymph nodes may result from reactivation of quiescent disease present in the nodes over many years. Biopsy and culture are particularly important in older people to differentiate tuberculous lymphadenopathy from that due to malignant disease.

144 Tuberculous meningitis – histology. If large numbers of tubercle bacilli escape into the bloodstream, meningitis may form part of a generalised tuberculosis; if small numbers are released, they may lodge in the brain forming a tuberculoma, which may subsequently leak into the subarachnoid space and cause meningitis. Tuberculous meningitis is generally less abrupt than other forms of bacterial meningitis and frequently presents as a febrile illness of undetermined origin. Symptoms may be extremely varied. The cerebrospinal fluid contains lymphocytes, or a mixture of lymphocytes and polymorphonuclear cells. The protein level is increased and the sugar level characteristically low. Tubercle bacilli may be scanty and detected only on culture. The tuberculin test may be negative in about one-half of patients.

This brain section shows the typical appearance of tuberculous meningitis. There is a granulomatous reaction in the meninges with caseation, round cell infiltration and giant cell formation.

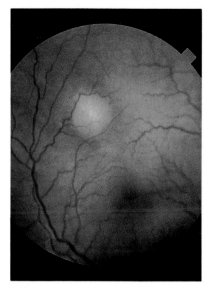
142

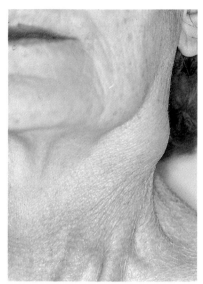
143

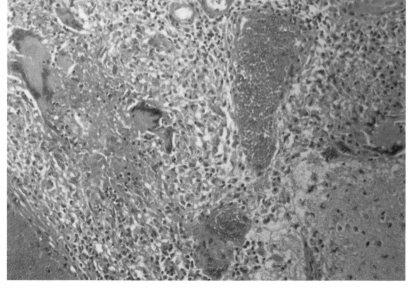
144

145 Acute tuberculous bronchopneumonia – chest radiograph. Post-primary infection may result from gradual extension of a caseous Ghon focus, may follow reactivation of a healed primary focus (especially if immunity wanes), or may be caused by fresh infection. It usually involves the lung apex and rarely affects regional lymph nodes. Spread is by local extension, via anatomical pathways such as the bronchial tree, or via the bloodstream after erosion of a blood vessel.

The disease is very variable and the extent of lung damage depends on the balance between exudation and fibrosis. On one hand there may be rapidly caseating pneumonia; on the other a chronic, well circumscribed cavity with much fibrosis. Pleural spread results in effusion or tuberculous empyema, but spread along the air passages produces tuberculous endobronchitis leading to cold abscess formation, bronchial obstruction, and bronchiectasis. Widespread fibroid tuberculosis with extensive destruction of lung tissue terminates in respiratory failure and cor pulmonale. If immunity is deficient the classical features of post-primary tuberculosis may be replaced by extensive local or generalised miliary spread.

The illness varies greatly and respiratory symptoms may be absent. Fever, unexplained weight loss and general deterioration in health may be the presenting features, while gastrointestinal symptoms such as loss of appetite and indigestion are not uncommon. The possibility of tuberculosis should always be considered in a patient with persistent cough, haemoptysis, or pneumonia not responding to antibiotic therapy. Except in advanced cases there may be no physical signs and chest radiographs should be taken in all suspected cases. The ultimate proof of the tuberculous nature of a lesion is detection of tubercle bacilli. Specimens of sputum, gastric washings, laryngeal or bronchial secretions should be examined for tubercle bacilli by direct fluorescence microscopy or by classic Ziehl-Neelsen technique, but culture is necessary to identify the organism and it may take 3–8 weeks to grow mycobacteria. Most pulmonary infections are caused by *M. tuberculosis*; a small proportion of patients yield atypical mycobacteria on culture.

This chest radiograph shows acute tuberculous bronchopneumonia with soft fluffy shadowing in both upper lobes.

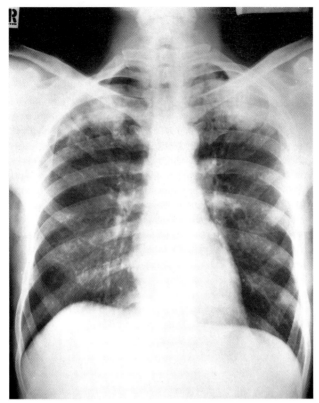

145

146 Chronic fibroid bronchopneumonia – chest radiograph. Active tuberculosis is associated with multiplication and invasion by tubercle bacilli with release of tuberculoproteins resulting in a cell-mediated immune response. The absorption of X-rays in the affected areas produces the soft fluffy shadowing that is very suggestive of active infection. However, it is important to stress that the presence or absence of active disease should be a microbiological, not a radiographic, judgement. Cavitation is common in post-primary pulmonary tuberculosis and healing of the diseased lung in immunocompetent patients gives rise to fibrosis and calcification. The presence of two or more of these features should suggest that the patient has had tuberculous infection at some time.

Chronic tuberculous pneumonia characteristically involves the apices. When cavitation is present the cavities are typically surrounded by areas of infiltration, resulting in dense homogeneous shadows on radiographic examination. Additional small patches of tuberculous bronchopneumonia may be situated peripherally and inferiorly to the main areas affected.

The chest radiograph opposite shows advanced fibroid tuberculosis with extensive fibrosis and calcification in the right lung. There is no cavitation.

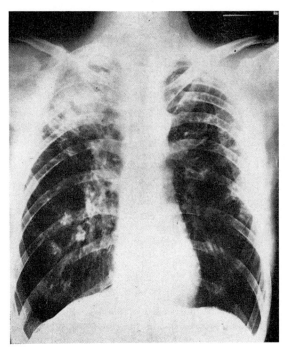

146

147   Aspergilloma – tomogram of lungs. Tuberculous cavities may be colonised by fungi, usually *Aspergillus fumigatus*. The typical appearance is of a rounded lesion, the 'fungus ball', above which there is an air halo. Clinical problems are unusual; occasionally massive haemoptysis may result. High levels of precipitating antibodies are found in the serum.

148   Renal tuberculosis – pyelogram. Tuberculosis of the urinary tract results from spread of the tubercle bacillus through the bloodstream. Although both kidneys may be infected, progressive disease is usually limited to one kidney and does not manifest clinically until 5–15 years have elapsed from primary infection. Hence, renal tuberculosis is typically a disease of adults rather than children. From the initial nidus in the cortex of the kidney, infection spreads to the renal papilla, where caseation is followed by the discharge of tubercle bacilli and spread of infection in the urine to the ureter and bladder. Subsequent healing by fibrosis may lead to strictures of the ureter and a small contracted bladder, causing obstruction to urinary flow and further kidney damage. Infection in males may spread from the urinary tract to the epididymis, seminal vesicles, and vas deferens, but rarely to the testis.

The disease commonly presents with increased frequency of micturition, dysuria or haematuria. Constitutional upset is unusual and patients may look surprisingly well. In the early stages of the disease examination of the urine may reveal a sterile pyuria; as the disease progresses proteinuria is a constant feature and is accompanied by varying haematuria. Acid-fast bacilli may be detected on microscopy but the diagnosis should be confirmed whenever possible by culture. Early changes on intravenous urography are those of bacterial pyelonephritis with blunting of the calyces and scarring of the cortex. Later there may be evidence of obstructive disease with strictures of the neck of the calyx or of the ureter, resulting in hydronephrosis. Gross destruction of the kidney as a result of severe back-pressure and caseation is referred to as autonephrectomy. Most patients are Mantoux-positive and half have concurrent active pulmonary disease.

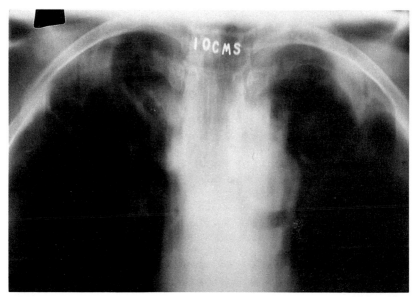

147

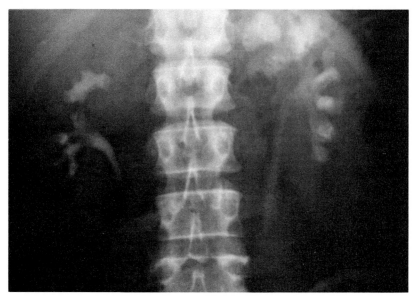

148

149 Tuberculous osteomyelitis – radiograph of spine. The spine is involved in half of the cases of tuberculous osteomyelitis. Infection is usually derived from the bloodstream although it may occasionally spread directly from nearby tissues. Typically the disease begins anteriorly in the vertebral bodies and leads to destruction of the intravertebral discs. In combination these two features produce the classical radiographic appearance with anterior wedging of two adjacent vertebrae and loss of disc space. When tuberculous pus forms, it usually spreads anteriorly to form a paraspinal abscess, which is confined by the paravertebral tissues and thus is forced to track away from the original focus.

Tuberculosis of other bones and joints is usually a combination of osteomyelitis and arthritis. The weight-bearing joints are commonly involved. Pain is usually the first symptom and may precede clinical or radiographic changes by several weeks. Radiographic examination may initially show soft tissue swelling. This is followed by osteoporosis, especially in the region of cartilages, and is accompanied by periosteal thickening and bone destruction around the joint. The final appearance is one of extensive bone destruction with periosteal thickening and abscess formation. Sinuses may develop and discharge pus. The radiological changes may take several weeks to appear but radioisotope bone scans may be positive at an earlier stage of infection. Biopsy may be required to confirm the diagnosis of bone tuberculosis.

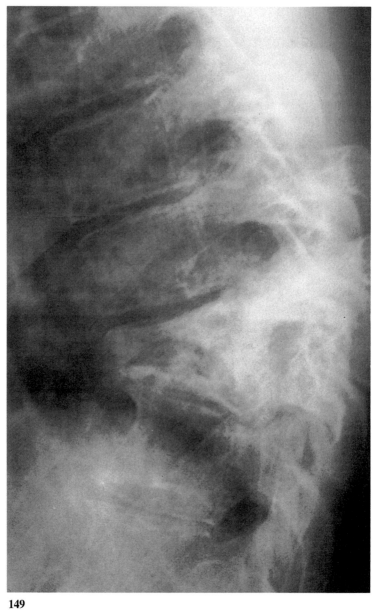

149

150   Tuberculosis of the skin. Tuberculosis may involve the skin in two main forms: localised infection, of which the commonest variety is lupus vulgaris, and the non-infectious tuberculids, in which the histological appearances are those of tuberculosis but tubercle bacilli cannot be demonstrated. In lupus vulgaris the bacillus is usually inoculated directly into the skin but it may spread from underlying lymph nodes, or via the lymphatics from the upper respiratory tract. A tuberculous granuloma forms at the entry point and the infection subsequently spreads via skin lymphatics in a circinate manner and gives rise to characteristic soft 'apple-jelly' nodules. As the disease advances, fresh nodules form and may coalesce to form a plaque, which may later ulcerate. Scarring is prominent and there is a tendency for nodules to recur in the scar tissue.

Other mycobacterial infections

151   Buruli ulcer. *Mycobacterium ulcerans (buruli)* is associated with slowly spreading indolent ulcers reported from country dwellers in Australia and Africa. The organism grows only between 30 and 35°C so, predictably, the cooler extremities of the body, especially the extensor surfaces, are most frequently affected.

A mobile nodule, 1–2 cm in diameter, forms initially at the site of infection. This quickly breaks down to produce a chronic, usually painless, cutaneous ulcer, which may extend to involve a very large area. The centre of the ulcer is necrotic and does not show caseation. Most of the organisms are present in the edge of the ulcer. Usually there is no enlargement of regional lymph nodes or systemic upset.

152   Aquarium granuloma. Aquarium (or swimming-pool) granuloma is caused by a marine mycobacterium, *Mycobacterium marinum (balnei)*, which has an optimum growth temperature of 30–33°C. Human infection is usually acquired directly from contaminated water but may occasionally result from direct inoculation as a result of trauma. After 2–8 weeks' incubation, papules develop at the implantation site. These enlarge progressively, undergo suppuration and eventually ulcerate. The sites usually affected are superficial and on the extremities, where the cooler temperature favours the organism. Although the lesions would eventually heal spontaneously, the process is accelerated by appropriate treatment.

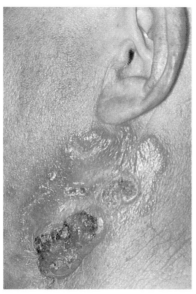

150

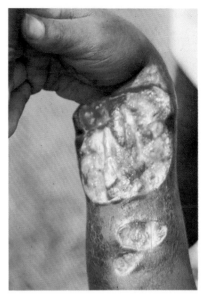

151

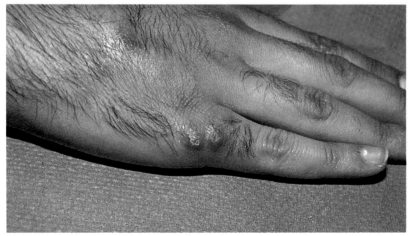

152

Leprosy

Leprosy is caused by *Mycobacterium leprae*, and man is the only natural host. The disease is found mainly in the tropics and subtropics. Close and continuous household contact is necessary for spread, and infection is usually derived from the nasal discharges of an infectious patient. Most infected people do not develop the disease; in those who do, the pattern of disease exhibits a spectrum from the tuberculoid, showing notable delayed hypersensitivity, to the lepromatous, in which there is virtually no cellular reaction by the host.

153   Organism – *Mycobacterium leprae*. This is a slender acid-fast bacillus, which has not been cultured on media or in tissue culture, but grows exceedingly slowly in the footpads of mice and armadillos. It replicates with a doubling time of about 13 days, and is an obligate intracellular parasite found in macrophages. The large number of organisms in this section of skin suggests that the patient had lepromatous leprosy.

154   Histology. The Schwann cells of peripheral nerves, being phagocytic, may contain bacteria. When there is a host response a granuloma is formed, consisting of epithelioid cells and giant cells surrounded by lymphocytes. As a result, the nerve may be compressed and damaged. Depending on the individual nerve this may result in motor or sensory disturbance, or both.

155   Lepromin reaction at 4 weeks. The lepromin reaction is a skin reaction observed after the intradermal injection of an extract of leprosy bacilli. It is of delayed hypersensitivity type but differs from the tuberculin reaction in that it is seen after several weeks rather than 48 hours. It is strongly positive in patients with tuberculoid leprosy and negative in those towards and at the lepromatous end of the spectrum.

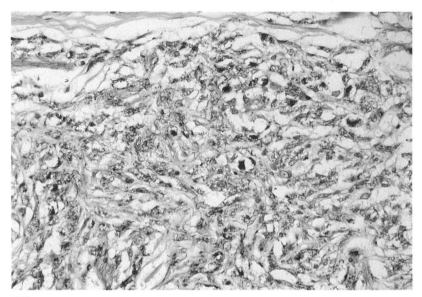

153

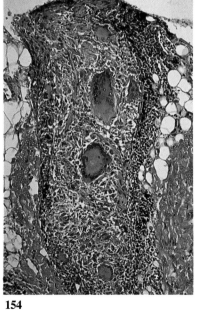

154

155

156 Appearance of face. The leonine facies is characteristic of lepromatous leprosy. The skin is thickened and ridged, the nose widened, and the ear lobes also thickened. Bacilli are readily found in large numbers in skin smears and also in the nodules shown here.

157 Erythema nodosum leprosum (ENL). Patients with lepromatous leprosy often suffer from ENL. The eruption is painful and consists of multiple reddened cutaneous nodules. It may be accompanied by constitutional upset, proteinuria, and orchitis. The incidence and severity of attacks vary greatly between patients, and may be precipitated by a variety of circumstances, including emotional factors. The underlying pathology is thought to be a vasculitis secondary to immune complex deposition.

158 'Upgrading' reaction. Patients whose disease is not at the two extremes of the spectrum may move their position in the spectrum according to the response to the organisms. Here, a patient towards the lepromatous end is showing more response than previously and is moving away from the lepromatous end in an upgrading reaction. Clinically this is seen as areas of erythema. Although this reaction may be considered as protective in nature, the increased cellular response may result in nerve compression and an increase in neurological findings.

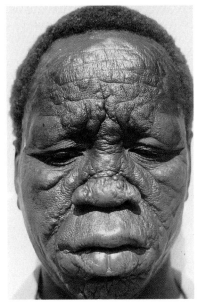

156

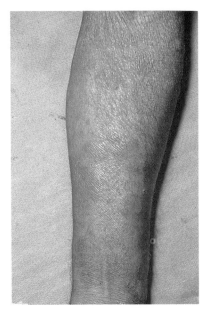

157

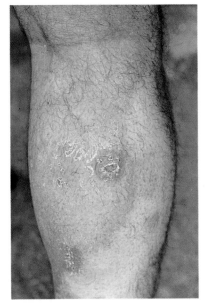

158

159   Tuberculoid leprosy. This patient is categorised towards the tuberculoid end of the immunological spectrum. Skin lesions are relatively few, asymmetrical, raised, anaesthetic, and do not sweat. Organisms are very scanty. Histologically the lesion is a granuloma; the lepromin test is strongly positive.

160   Nerve infection. In some patients the disease is purely neural and no skin lesions are seen. In this patient the radial nerve is affected, causing wrist drop and anaesthesia of the thumb.

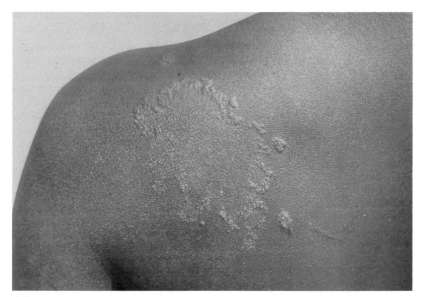

159

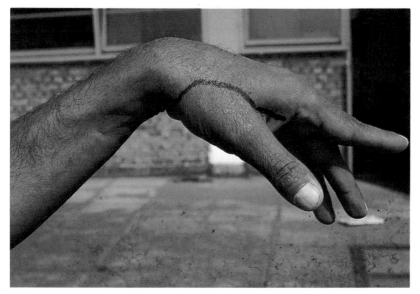

160

161 Claw hand. Claw hand is a characteristic feature of leprosy, especially in those patients categorised in the middle of the spectrum with borderline disease. The ulnar nerve is affected; patients are unable to flex the metacarpophalangeal joints, and there is prominent wasting of the thenar and hypothenar eminences. The deformity may be aggravated by the subsequent contractures. Sensory loss is present in the ulnar distribution.

162 Ulcers. Ulcers of the feet are common in leprosy. They may be perforating ulcers of the sole, similar to those seen in diabetes, or round the ankle, as seen here. Because of anaesthesia the foot is vulnerable to damage from prolonged pressure, burns, or general injuries. The ulcers are slow to heal and tend to break down; they may be associated with considerable loss of tissue, scarring, and deformity.

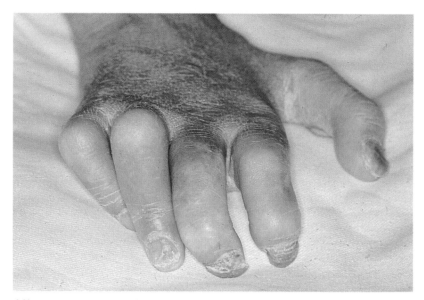

161

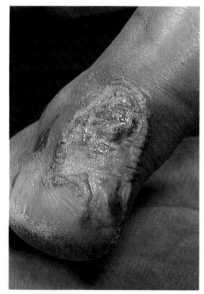

162

Tetanus

163 *Clostridium tetani* – **negative stain with nigrosin.** The tetanus bacillus is ubiquitous, being present in soil and dust, though the degree of contamination varies from district to district. It is frequently found in the intestinal tract of animals and sometimes humans. It is a Gram-positive rod measuring 2·5 μm in length and is a strict anaerobe. It forms spherical terminal spores, highly resistant to heat and disinfectants.

Tetanus bacilli may be spread by direct introduction of spores by penetrating injury, direct contamination of wounds, burns and umbilical stumps by dust or faeces, or contaminated syringes used by drug addicts. Tetanus does not spread from person to person. The spores germinate when introduced into tissues with low oxygen tension, such as wounds with necrotic tissue including those with concomitant contamination with aerobic bacteria. The vegetative bacilli growing in the wound subsequently produce a potent exotoxin with a special affinity for nervous tissue. The toxin is absorbed by local motor nerve endings and is conveyed to the nervous system, where it disturbs the regulation of reflex arcs and abolishes reciprocal innervation. Consequently, afferent stimuli produce an exaggerated response. The organism itself is not invasive.

164 Trismus. Difficulty in opening the mouth due to increased tone in the masseters is usually the first evidence of tetanus. At this early stage mumps may be suspected, but hypertonus can usually be detected in muscles elsewhere, and the salivary glands are not swollen. Lockjaw, the old name for tetanus, aptly describes the condition.

Pain and stiffness in the neck and back may simulate meningitis, but the correct diagnosis becomes apparent as the disease advances.

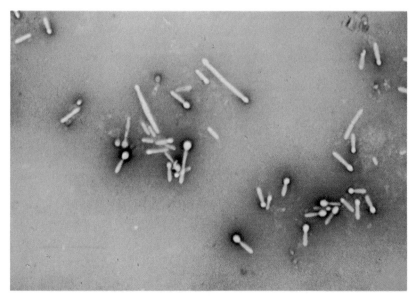

163

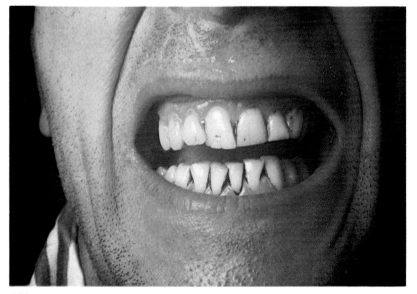

164

165 Risus sardonicus. Spasm of the facial muscles causes retraction of the angles of the mouth to expose the clenched teeth in a characteristic snarling grin.

166 Opisthotonus in a child. Tetanus toxin causes overactivity of motor nerve cells, resulting in muscle rigidity and spasm. Tonic rigidity is present in every case and persists throughout the illness. When the spinal muscles are severely affected opisthotonus results. In mild attacks the disease may be arrested at the stage of rigidity, and spasms do not develop.

If the disease advances spasms appear and become progressively more frequent and severe. With the onset of a convulsion the whole body is suddenly thrown into a violent spasm by the sustained contraction of all somatic muscles. The jaws are tightly clenched, the back arched, and the limbs are usually extended. Each paroxysm may be accompanied by muscle cramp so severe that the patient lies in dread of the next attack. Patients remain fully conscious throughout their terrifying ordeal.

167 Tetanus neonatorum. The umbilical stump may be infected by the use of non-sterile instruments or dressings, and this may lead to neonatal tetanus. Failure to suck is an early sign and is followed by hypertonus and muscle spasms. Despite treatment mortality rates may exceed 50%.

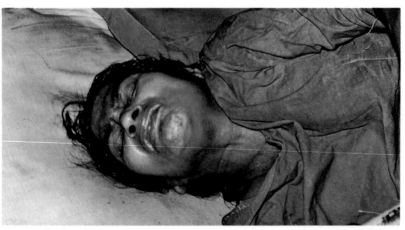

165

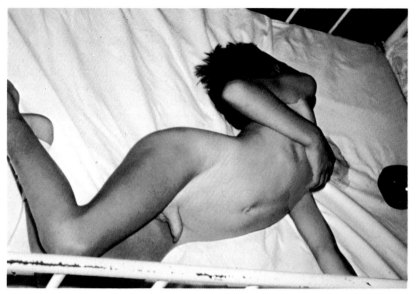

166

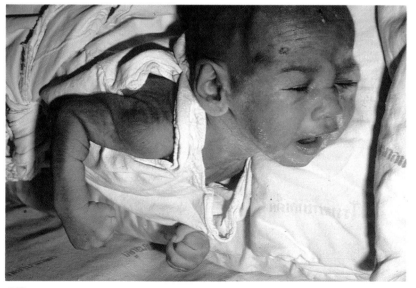

167

Anthrax

168 Smear from culture of anthrax bacilli (Gram stain). Anthrax is a world-wide zoonosis, endemic in areas where animal infection is common. The disease is caused by a bacillus that forms highly resistant spores on exposure to oxygen. In tropical countries, where climatic conditions favour rapid sporulation with heavy contamination of soil, anthrax is mainly spread from infected pasture, where spores may remain viable for many years. In temperate climates, where sporulation is less rapid and vegetative bacilli are readily destroyed by soil bacteria, contamination of pasture land is slight and infection is usually derived from imported animal products such as hair, hides, and bone meal. Sheep, goats, cattle, and horses are very susceptible. Person-to-person transmission has not been reported.

Bacillus anthracis is a non-motile, Gram-positive, spore-bearing rod, 4–10 μm in length, and is one of the largest of the pathogenic bacteria. In smears from infected animals the bacilli are encapsulated and lie singly or in short chains; in cultures on nutrient agar capsules are not formed and the organism is arranged in long strands. When exposed to oxygen it forms spores that are oval in shape with a double-layered outer membrane. *B. anthracis* is the only virulent pathogenic species in a genus of ubiquitious free-living bacilli.

169 Anthrax bacilli in pulmonary capillaries – Gram stain (× 880). Pulmonary anthrax (or wool-sorters' disease) is a rare condition in humans, acquired by inhaling anthrax spores in dust from contaminated wool or hair. The onset is abrupt and the illness follows a rapid course with frequent haemoptyses and acute respiratory distress culminating in death within 2 or 3 days.

On autopsy there is severe pulmonary oedema with widespread haemorrhagic bronchopneumonia. Large numbers of anthrax bacilli are present and are very conspicuous in Gram-stained preparations because of their large size and deep blue colour.

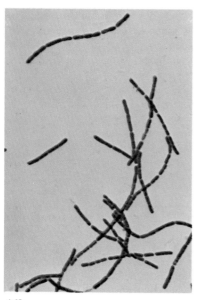

168

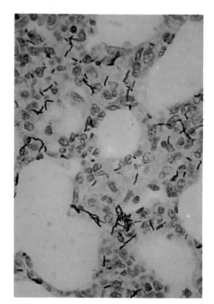

169

170 Cutaneous anthrax (malignant pustule) – early lesion on neck. The skin is involved in 98% of human infections, and lesions are found most frequently on exposed areas of the body. Infection may be acquired directly from animals, but is more commonly derived from hides, wool, hair, bonemeal, or other animal products.

Anthrax is an occupational disease of hide porters, caused by infected hides rubbing against the neck. An itchy papule develops at the site of entry and is surrounded within a day or two by a ring of haemorrhagic vesicles. Oedema is a striking feature of cutaneous anthrax, beginning round the original lesion and spreading extensively wherever the subcutaneous tissues are lax. The skin may retain its normal colour or become intensely red. Blood cultures may prove positive.

171 Anthrax lesion on the neck. As the lesion progresses the central area ulcerates and dries, forming a thick, leathery, dark scab. This later extends into the vesicular zone. The crust is firmly attached to the underlying tissues and gradually separates over a period of 2–3 weeks, leaving a deep ulcer which heals slowly with granulation tissue. The lesion is painless and pus seldom forms, except on the rare occasions of secondary infection. Before the introduction of antibiotics deaths from anthrax of the neck were much greater than from anthrax of the forehead.

Anthrax bacilli are numerous beneath the central necrotic area. Both the capsule of the organism and the exotoxin produced by the growing bacilli inhibit phagocytosis. Bacteraemia may follow primary infection at any site.

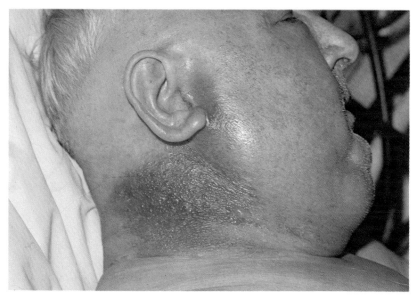

170

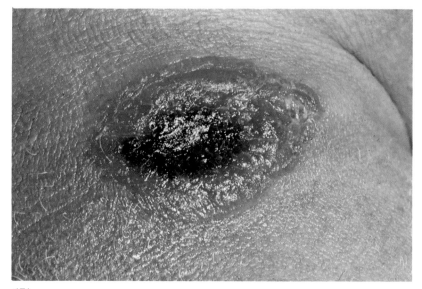

171

172 Anthrax of the forearm. This condition may affect butchers handling infected carcasses, or gardeners using contaminated bonemeal. Oedema may be slight. The eschar in the illustration is just beginning to separate.

173 Anthrax of the back. The lower limbs and trunk are less commonly affected, being involved in only 1.9% of cases. The patient opposite worked in a factory manufacturing paint brushes. She developed a large lesion over her left scapula, but there was very little constitutional disturbance. By the time the photograph was taken the vesicles had ruptured and had been incorporated in the eschar, which was firmly adherent.

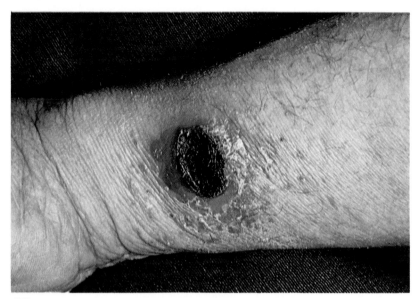

172

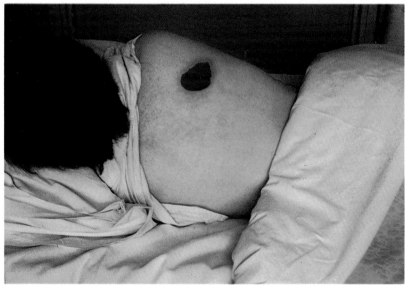

173

Leptospirosis

174 Smear from culture of *Leptospira icterohaemorrhagiae* (silver impregnation stain). The genus *Leptospira* includes two main species: *L. interrogens* and *L. biflexia*. Both species contain many serotypes (serovars), some of which are pathogenic, and others saprophytic. Parasitic leptospires are indistinguishable from one another morphologically or culturally but can be classified serologically. More than 50 serotypes have already been identified. Leptospires are about 7–14 μm long and have a closely coiled body with hooked ends. On electron microscopy the cytoplasm is seen to be wound round a single, straight and stiff axostyle. The organism is actively motile. It is an aerobe, and parasitic strains grow readily on fluid culture medium containing animal serum.

Leptospirosis is a zoonosis affecting rodents, dogs, cats, pigs and cattle. Leptospires may cause little harm to the primary host, where they colonise the renal tubules and are shed in large numbers in the urine. Humans and susceptible animals may be infected indirectly by water or articles contaminated by such urine. The organism enters through minor breaches in the skin or mucosa. Farm workers and sewage workers are at special risk.

175 Section of liver showing leptospires (silver impregnation stain). There is no obvious reaction at the portal of entry, and the organisms quickly enter the bloodstream. When death occurs during the first week of illness leptospires can be found in many tissues but subsequently they are most easily detected in the kidneys. They are best demonstrated by fluorescent antibody technique.

There is a striking contrast between the depth of jaundice in severe cases of leptospirosis and the histological changes in the liver. Damage to the liver cells is much less severe than in viral hepatitis, and the serum transaminase activity is often only slightly increased. Cholestasis is the most prominent feature. In post-mortem preparations the parenchymal cells are seen to be separated from each other, and there is a high incidence of mitotic figures.

In this section, stained by Levaditi's silver impregnation method, a large number of leptospires with characteristic closely wound spirals can be seen scattered between the liver cells. (Arrow = leptospire.)

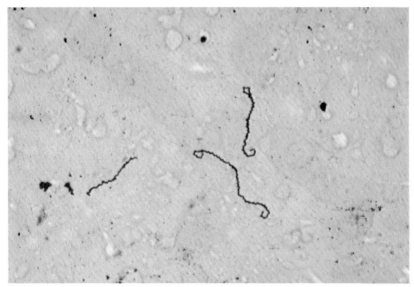

174

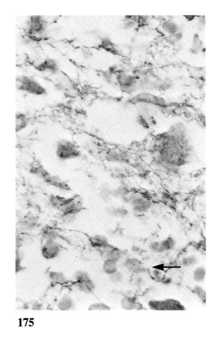

175

176 Suffusion of conjunctivas. Leptospirosis in humans is associated with a wide range of clinical syndromes, including classic Weil's disease, aseptic meningitis, influenza-like illness, and unexplained fever. The onset is abrupt with shivering followed by fever. Headache, myalgia and arthralgia are common features. Conjunctival suffusion is often present and may be accompanied by photophobia. Prostration tends to be severe and disproportionate to the physical signs.

177 Close-up of eye in canicola fever. Human beings usually develop canicola fever through contact with pig or dog urine containing *L. canicola*, although the leptospire is sometimes found in other animals. Severe and intractable headache is an outstanding and distressing symptom. An aseptic form of meningitis is present in 75% of patients. Roughly 20% have jaundice or evidence of renal damage. Nearly 50% have injection of the conjunctivae.

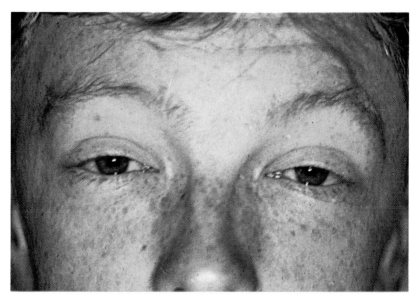

176

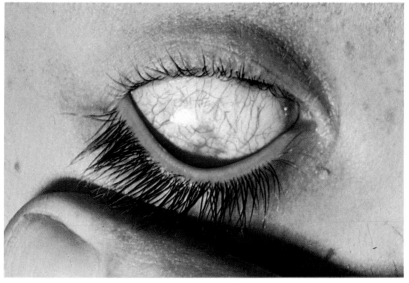

177

178   Severe Weil's disease. Weil's disease is a severe form of leptospirosis with both hepatic and renal damage. It is commonly caused by *L. icterohaemorrhagiae* derived from rats, but other serotypes have been incriminated. The syndrome is comparatively rare, occurring in roughly 15% of leptospiral infections in humans. Even with this most virulent serotype, mild or inapparent infections are not uncommon.

The first week of illness is dominated by fever, headache, severe debility, and muscular pains. Nausea and vomiting may be accompanied by haematemesis, and abdominal pain may be so severe that a surgical emergency is suspected. Jaundice may be the earliest sign but may not develop until the end of the first week. At the same time haemorrhages may appear in the skin and mucous membranes and, if profuse, indicate an unfavourable prognosis. The second week is critical. Jaundice deepens, haemorrhages increase, and renal failure develops. Most deaths take place at this stage from renal failure and some lives may be saved by effective dialysis. During the third week the illness abates, renal function improves, and jaundice lessens. Eventually full renal and hepatic function are restored.

179   The face in Weil's disease. Haemorrhages are common in severely ill patients with jaundice and renal failure. Petechiae or ecchymoses may be found in skin, conjunctivae, or mucous membranes. Epistaxis may be a presenting feature, and there may be profuse bleeding into the bowel during the second week. Mild haemoptysis is not unusual.

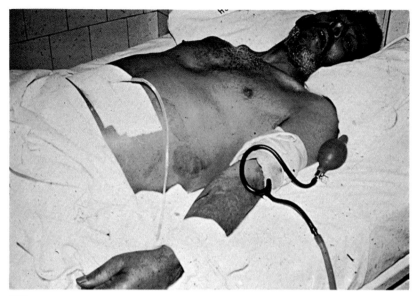

178

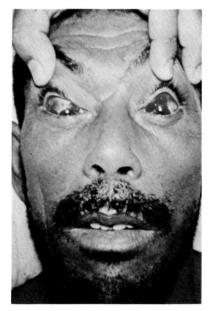

179

Gonorrhoea

Gonorrhoea is caused by *Neisseria gonorrhoeae*, an infection confined to humans. In adults it is transmitted by sexual contact; in children by non-sexual contact or by fomites. Gonorrhoea in adults may manifest as local infection of the urogenital tract, rectum, conjunctiva or oropharynx, or generalised infection of the skin, joints, meninges, and endocardium. Transmission from the mother during delivery may result in acute conjunctivitis; contamination of flannels and towels may cause acute vulvovaginitis in young girls.

180 Smear of pus (Gram stain). *Neisseria gonorrhoeae* is a Gram-negative bacterium, usually sensitive to human serum and readily ingested by neutrophil polymorphonuclear leucocytes, as seen in this smear stained with Gram stain, where they appear as intracellular diplococci. They have fastidious growth requirements.

181 Urethritis. This is the most common presentation of gonorrhoea in men. A purulent urethral discharge appears within a few days after exposure and is associated with dysuria. Untreated this will often last for many weeks before clearing spontaneously. The persistent inflammation predisposes to urethral stricture. Gonococcal urethritis is clinically indistinguishable from non-gonococcal urethritis caused by chlamydia, but can be differentiated by examination of a urethral smear. Painful lymphadenitis is present in 15% of cases. Proctitis may be the presenting feature in homosexuals.

182 Cervicitis. Symptoms are absent in 80% of women infected with the gonoccocus. An infected cervix may have a normal appearance with mucoid discharge or may be inflamed with mucopurulent or profuse purulent discharge. The urethra or rectum may be infected from the vaginal discharge. Pelvic spread may result in endometritis, salpingitis, or peritonitis.

183 Bartholin's abscess. A more dramatic presentation in women is infection of Bartholin's gland. The lymphadenitis is usually unilateral and may progress to form abscesses. Skene's glands may also be affected.

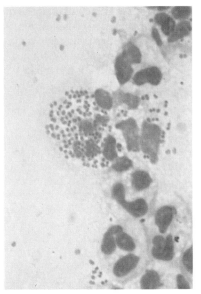

180

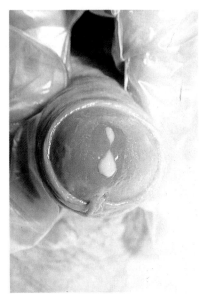

181

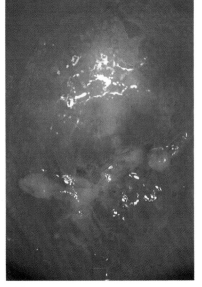

182

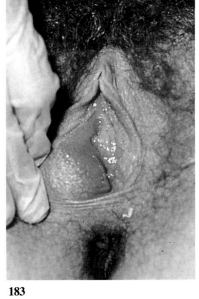

183

184 Gonorrhoea – skin lesions. Disseminated infection is caused by strains of gonococci resistant to serum and accounts for 2% of all gonococcal infection. It is more common in women. Bacteraemia may lead to septic arthritis, tenosynovitis, meningitis, endocarditis, or skin lesions. Skin lesions are the most common feature and consist of a sparse rash over the limbs, sparing the face and trunk.

185 Gonorrhoea – close-up of skin lesion. The most characteristic lesion is a pustule on an erythematous base. Slight fever is common. Some patients may have no constitutional upset; others may be very ill with a high fever.

186 Gonorrhoea – close-up of skin lesion. The skin lesions vary and may consist of macules, papules, pustules, haemorrhagic bullae, or necrotic lesions as shown here. The organism is seldom grown from the skin lesions but may be cultured from blood or purulent joint effusions. Most patients have migratory arthralgia during the first week, mainly affecting the large joints. In some cases this will progress to septic arthritis. Tenosynovitis is found in about 25% of cases.

187 Conjunctivitis. Ophthalmia may result from direct contact with an infected birth canal. It follows 2–5 days after birth and may cause septicaemia. Transfer of infection from discharges elsewhere may cause conjunctivitis in adults. Young girls living in overcrowded conditions are very susceptible to gonococcal vulvovaginitis spread by moist articles such as flannels or towels. Infection is very seldom spread by fomites to adults.

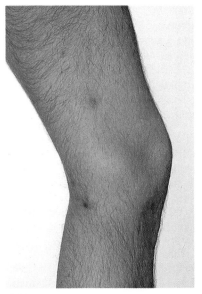

184

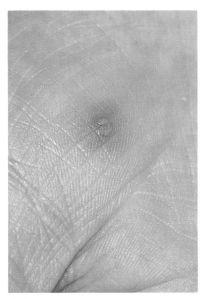

185

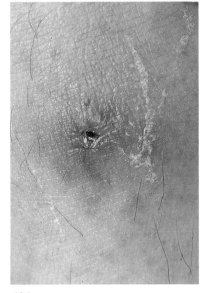

186

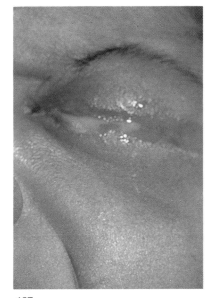

187

Chlamydial infection

Chlamydia are intracellular parasites, whose genome contains both DNA and RNA. They are considered to be specialised bacteria with a complex form of replication ending in binary fission, and can be divided into two groups sharing a complement-fixing antigen. *Chlamydia trachomatis* (group A) is responsible for genital infections, conjunctivitis at any age and pneumonitis in infancy; *Chlamydia psittaci* (group B) causes ornithosis.

188   Chlamydial infection – conjunctival smear. Conjunctival scrapings from patients with neonatal inclusion conjunctivitis, when stained by Giemsa's method, may show intracytoplasmic basophilic inclusion bodies. The technique is less sensitive in adult inclusion conjunctivitis, and of little or no value in genital infection. Tissue cultures, using pretreated cells, such as McCoy, are more reliable. Humoral antibody may be detected by immunofluorescence, but the results of serological tests must be interpreted with caution.

189   Conjunctivitis in a newborn baby. Infection of the eye from the mother's cervix at the time of birth may result in inclusion conjunctivitis of the newborn. A mucopurulent conjunctivitis develops within 2 weeks of birth and may affect one or both eyes. There are no distinguishing features. The acute stage settles after 2 weeks or so, but the eye may take several months to return to normal and the disease may progress to mild trachoma.

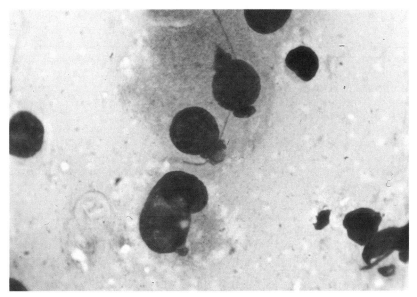

188

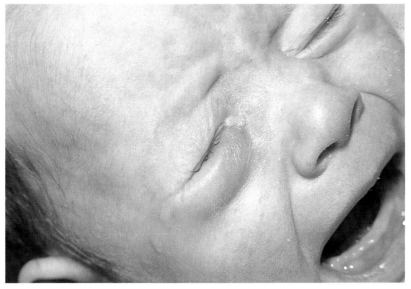

189

190 Conjunctivitis in an adult. Inclusion conjunctivitis in adults also has an acute onset and is accompanied by mucopurulent discharge, conjunctival follicles and superficial punctate keratitis. The follicles are always more prominent in the lower than the upper lid, and appear as rounded swellings, 1–2 mm in diameter, which are formed by lymphocytic foci in the subepithelial adenoid layer. Healing takes place slowly over a period of 1–2 years.

191 Trachoma. Trachoma is also caused by TRIC or non-LGV strains of *Chlamydia trachomatis*. The disease is endemic in many parts of the world where people are crowded together under conditions of poor hygiene. Infection is transmitted by conjunctival secretions, which are transferred on fingers or towels and, above all, by flies. The onset is usually subacute and the course is determined by the presence or absence of secondary infection. The conjunctiva is inflamed and follicles appear in the fornices. They spread over the palpebral conjunctiva but rarely on to the bulbar conjunctiva, and may measure up to 5 mm in diameter. Trachomatous infiltration may extend deeply into the subepithelial tissues of the palpebral conjunctiva. The cornea is affected at an early stage with a superficial keratitis, which is most marked in the upper part. As the disease progresses the conjunctiva becomes scarred and pannus develops, with cloudiness and vascularisation of the cornea.

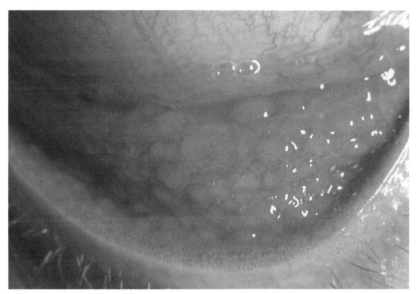

190

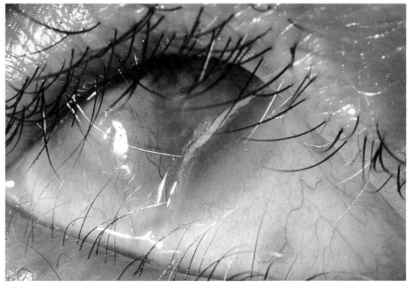

191

192　Urethritis. *Chlamydia trachomatis* may be isolated from the urethra in up to 5% of symptomless men, 20% of men with gonorrhoea, and 30–50% of men with non-specific urethritis. Chlamydial urethritis is clinically indistinguishable from gonococcal urethritis, though it tends to be milder. Chlamydial infection is also associated with epididymitis and with Reiter's disease.

193　Cervicitis. Chlamydial infections are common in women: the organism has been detected in up to 5% of healthy women, and up to 60% of women with gonorrhoea. Chlamydial cervicitis is accompanied by mucopurulent discharge from the os, and the cervix is reddened and oedematous. Chlamydia is responsible for some cases of salpingitis and proctitis in women. Infection acquired at birth may give rise to inclusion conjunctivitis in the newborn baby, or pneumonitis in the infant.

194　Lymphogranuloma venereum. This sexually transmitted disease is caused by the LGV strain of *Chlamydia trachomatis*. After an incubation period of 1–3 weeks a primary lesion may be detected on the genitals in about 10% of patients. This consists of a small papule or vesicle, which may ulcerate, but heals within a few days without leaving a scar.

After 2–10 weeks the patient enters the secondary stage, with painful swelling of the regional lymph nodes. This is occasionally accompanied by constitutional disturbance, with fever, headache and arthralgia. As the disease progresses the lymph nodes become matted and attached to the overlying skin, which is reddened. The buboes may suppurate and discharge through sinuses on to the surface of the skin, vagina or bowel.

The disease may resolve after 3–4 months, or may advance to the third stage, with strictures of the urethra, vagina or rectum. Fistulas or perirectal abscesses may prove troublesome and lymphatic obstruction may result in chronic oedema with enlargement of the penis or vulva.

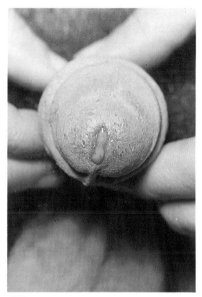

192

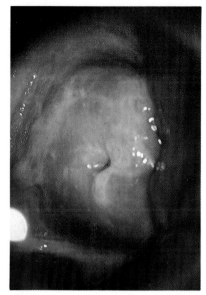

193

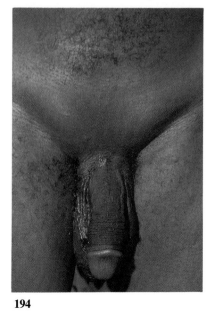

194

195 Ornithosis. This is a worldwide zoonosis caused by *Chlamydia psittaci.* Infection is common in humans occupationally exposed to psittacine birds in pet shops and aviaries, and other birds in turkey and duck processing plants. Infection is rarely transmitted from humans.

Much infection is subclinical or mild, resembling influenza. Severe attacks begin with an influenza-like illness. During the first week the patient has a high fever with relative bradycardia and possible gastrointestinal disturbance with diarrhoea. A dry cough may be present, but there are few chest signs. Evidence of consolidation may appear during the second week, and the extent of the pneumonia on radiological examination is disproportionate to the physical signs. The radiographic appearances are not diagnostic. The erythrocyte sedimentation rate tends to be notably increased, and the diagnosis is confirmed by serological tests. The illness subsides after 7–14 days, but convalescence tends to be protracted, and radiological clearance may take several weeks.

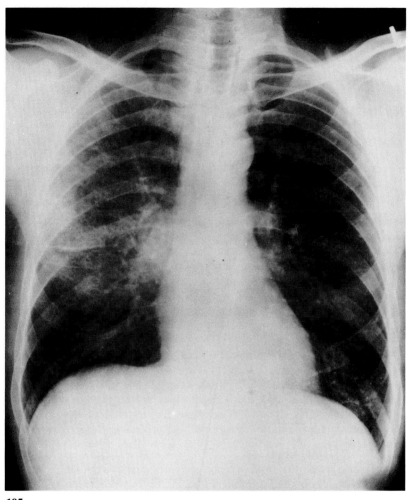

195

Syphilis

Syphilis is caused by the spirochaete *Treponema pallidum*. Acquired infection is almost entirely transmitted by sexual contact; congenital infection often comes from a mother who has been infected during or shortly before pregnancy. The incidence of syphilis has greatly declined since the introduction of antibiotics.

196 *Treponema pallidum* – **dark-ground illumination.** *Treponema pallidum* is a slender spirochaete about 10 μm in length with roughly ten turns to its spiral. It has an undulating movement and rotates about its long axis. It is sensitive to drying and dies rapidly above 42°C but can survive for some days at 4°C. It cannot be seen by ordinary microscopy but is best seen by dark-field illumination as shown here; it can be stained by silver in tissue sections. It is a human parasite and is indistinguishable morphologically or serologically from treponemes causing yaws, pinta or bejel.

197 Primary syphilis – chancre in a male. The primary lesion of syphilis, the chancre, appears within 2–4 weeks of infection. In heterosexual men this is most commonly found on the glans penis or in the sulcus, and less commonly on the penile shaft. The chancre is indurated but is not tender, and is frequently associated with enlarged but painless inguinal lymph nodes. Dark-field preparations are made from serum exuded from the chancre. Serological tests do not become positive for 3–4 weeks.

198 Primary syphilis – chancre in a female. Classically, the chancre appears after an incubation period of 21–35 days (extremes 9–90 days) as a single lesion in 50% of cases. It evolves rapidly from a macule to a papule, which erodes and forms a round, painless ulcer with a clean surface and surrounding hard induration. It heals within 3–10 weeks, leaving a thin atrophic scar in some cases. Vulval lesions may be readily recognised, but cervical lesions are commonly overlooked.

199 Primary syphilis – anal chancre. In homosexual men the anus is a major site for the primary lesion. Anal lesions may also be found in women, and mouth lesions occur in both sexes.

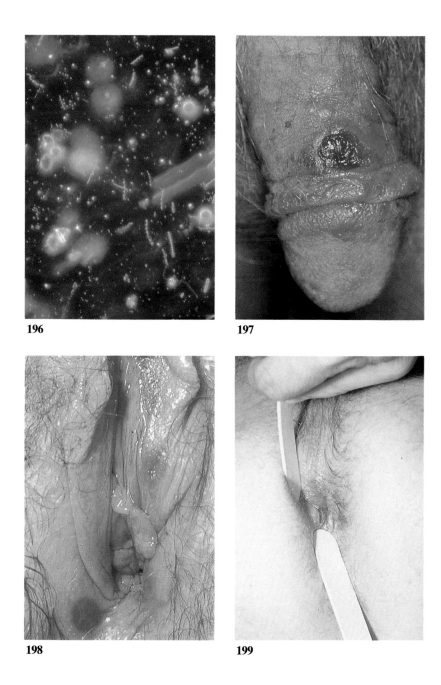

196

197

198

199

200 Secondary syphilis – rash. A rash is the presenting feature in 70% of cases and usually appears 6–8 weeks after infection, when the primary lesion is declining or has healed. It may be accompanied by general symptoms of fever, headache, malaise and arthralgia, and associated with mucous patches, lymphadenitis and meningitis. The rash varies greatly in intensity and appearance. It usually appears first on the trunk and proximal parts of the limbs as discrete pinkish macules, which may evolve into red papules. The lesions do not itch and persist for 4–8 weeks.

201 Secondary syphilis – rash. Sometimes the rash may consist of fewer, larger, darker red papules.

202 Secondary syphilis – close-up of rash. In a few patients the rash may finally become pustular and form crusts. Lesions of different type may be found on the same patient. Vesicular rashes are not a feature of secondary syphilis.

203 Secondary syphilis rash. The rash may extend to cover the whole body, including the palms and soles. This distribution should suggest possible secondary syphilis. Involvement of hair follicles may result in patchy alopecia.

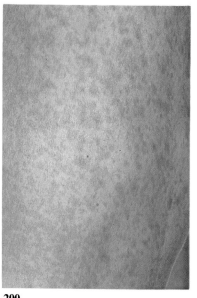

200

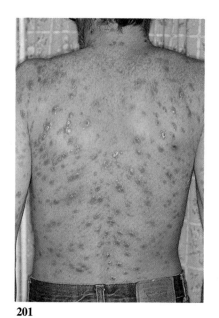

201

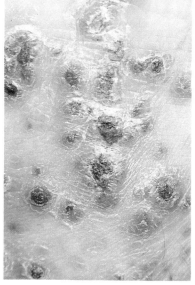

202

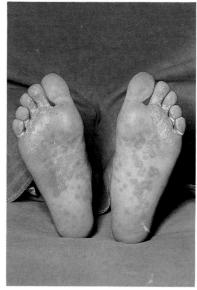

203

204 Secondary syphilis – mucosal lesions. Lesions, termed mucous patches, may also be present on the surface of the mucous membranes of the mouth, pharynx, larynx, and genitals. They usually take the form of superficial erosions but papules may occasionally be seen. The patches are round, oval or serpiginous in outline and may be dull red in colour or covered with a greyish membrane. The serpiginous lesions have been termed snail-track ulcers. Saliva from such patients is highly infectious.

When the secondary stage subsides the patient enters the stage of latent syphilis. There is no clinical evidence of active disease, but serological tests remain positive. Before the introduction of penicillin for the treatment of syphilis, between 10 and 20% of patients progressed to the tertiary stage.

205 Tertiary syphilis – gumma. The basic lesion of tertiary syphilis is a chronic granuloma, known as gumma. It tends to be localised, asymmetrical in distribution, and destructive in character. A gumma may affect any part of the body. Sometimes a solitary gumma may appear in the subcutaneous tissues, increasing in size before breaking down to form a gummatous ulcer. Such an ulcer is painless and has a characteristic appearance. It is roughly circular, with sharply defined 'punched out' edges and an indurated base. A slough of necrotic tissue, like a piece of wash-leather, initially occupies the crater and is firmly adherent. Later, it separates leaving pale granulations. Spirochaetes cannot be detected in the lesion.

206 Tertiary syphilis – chest radiograph, showing aneurysm. Cardiovascular disease may develop 10–30 years after infection and is accompanied by neurosyphilis in about 30% of cases. Vasculitis affecting the vasa vasorum of the aorta results in loss of elastic tissue and subsequent dilatation of the artery. If the root of the aorta is affected the aortic ring becomes dilated, causing aortic incompetence.

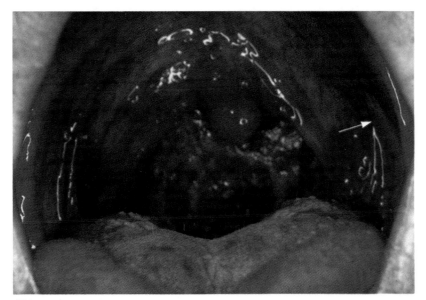

204

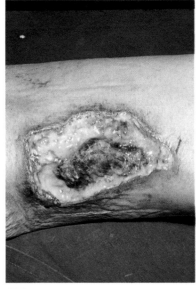

205

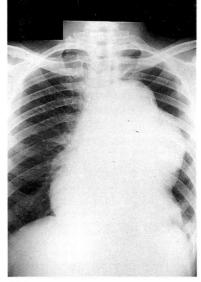

206

177

207 Congenital syphilis – histology of liver (silver impregnation stain).
Congenital syphilis is now extremely rare in developed countries. The clinical course is very variable and in many cases there may be no obvious clinical signs. One of the earliest features may be a mucopurulent nasal discharge, which may persist for many months and is known as the 'snuffles'. Skin eruptions are common during the first 2 years of life, and there may be evidence of damage to many structures, including mucous membranes, bones, and teeth. The liver may be severely affected and in fatal cases large numbers of spirochaetes may be present. (Arrows point to organism.)

208 Congenital syphilis – early manifestations. The rash in congenital syphilis is most commonly maculopapular and may be followed by extensive sloughing of the epithelium on the palms and soles and around the mouth and anus. Pemphigoid lesions may be found in congenital syphilis but rarely in acquired syphilis. The skin lesions are teeming with treponema.

The early lesions heal and after a latent period the late features appear. These include damage to teeth, bones, eyes and auditory nerve, as well as gummas and neurosyphilis.

209 Radiograph of tibia and fibula in the late form of syphilitic periostitis.
Widespread bone disease is very common in young children with congenital syphilis and may present as osteochondritis, periostitis, or osteitis and osteomyelitis, particularly affecting the long bones and the skull. This early disease may be detected at any time from birth to the age of 3–4 years and usually resolves spontaneously.

Bone disease may reappear between the ages of 5 and 15 years. This late form is usually very resistant to treatment and may persist indefinitely. The radiological appearances in syphilitic, tuberculous and chronic pyogenic bone disease are very similar, and other factors must be taken into consideration when making a diagnosis. In the juvenile form of syphilitic periostitis or osteitis new bone may be deposited in lamellated layers parallel to the shaft or else on the convexity of the shaft. The tibia is commonly affected, and thickening of the anterior aspect of the proximal half of the bone may produce the appearance of sabre shin or tibia.

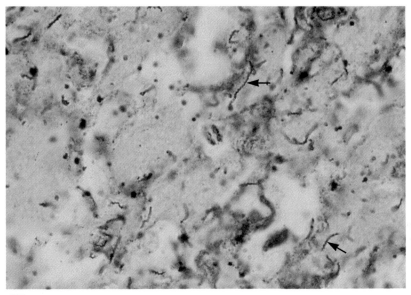

207

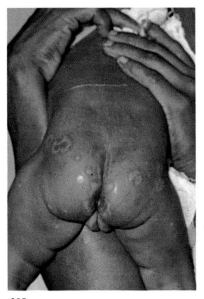

208

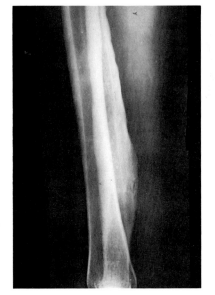

209

Donovanosis

Donovanosis, granuloma inguinale, and granuloma venereum are names given to the disease produced by *Calymmatobacterium granulomatis*, a Gram-negative encapsulated bacterium, whose relation to other organisms is uncertain. Infection is usually transmitted by sexual contact, but this is not exclusive, as young children may be affected. It is more common in tropical parts of the world.

210 Donovanosis – organism. This is characteristically found in large mononuclear cells and can be demonstrated as deeply staining Donovan bodies in smudge smears made from the lesions. In this smear the preparation was made from the penile lesion. The organism is difficult to culture on artificial media.

211 Donovanosis – lesions. The disease is usually confined to the genitals, but other sites may be affected. In men the penis is the common site, in women the labia. The primary lesion is an indurated nodule, which becomes ulcerated. Individual lesions may coalesce to form enlarging areas of ulceration, and autoinfection may occur. In this patient from Papua New Guinea spread of infection to the inguinal lymph nodes from the initial penile lesion has resulted in extensive ulceration in the groins. Secondary infection may cause further damage and scarring may lead to deformity.

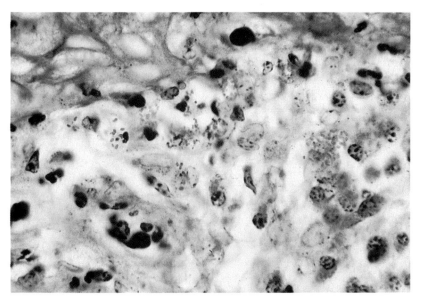

210

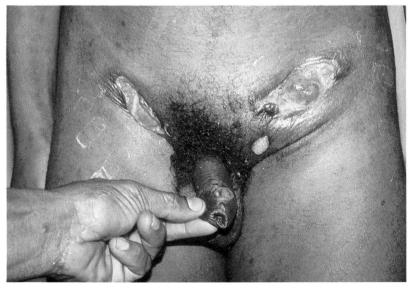

211

Chancroid

Chancroid is a sexually transmitted disease caused by the Gram-negative cocco-bacillus *Haemophilus ducreyi*. As with a number of sexually transmitted diseases, it is more commonly recognised in men than women. The infection is worldwide in distribution and is especially common where social, economic, and hygienic conditions are poor.

Lesions are usually confined to the genitalia and perianal region, with secondary lesions in the inguinal lymph nodes. The initial lesion is a tender papule, which becomes pustular and then erodes to form a non-indurated and painful ulcer. This may coalesce with other lesions, and secondary infection may result in further destruction.

212   Genital lesions in chancroid. Here the penile lesions are associated with greatly enlarged inguinal glands. The lymphadenitis is usually unilateral. The swelling is painful and may rupture to leave a discharging sinus. The penile lesions may be difficult to distinguish from those of granuloma inguinale (Donovanosis). They may also be confused with the primary lesion of syphilis, but can be differentiated by the presence of pain and absence of induration. The two infections coexist in up to 10% of patients, so the possibility of syphilis should always be considered. The diagnosis of chancroid may be confirmed by finding the organism in smears or by culture.

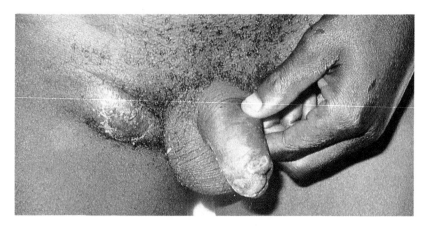

212

VIRUS INFECTIONS

Herpesvirus group

Members of this group cause important infections in both humans and animals. Those associated with human disease include:

- *Herpesvirus varicellae/zoster* – the cause of chickenpox and herpes zoster.
- Herpes simplex virus.
- *Herpesvirus simiae* – a rare cause of encephalitis in humans.
- Cytomegalovirus – benign lymphadenitis and other syndromes.
- Epstein–Barr virus – associated with infectious mononucleosis and neoplastic disease.

The herpesviruses are relatively large, 120–180 nm, with a central capsid containing DNA and an outer membrane derived from the host cell. They are ether sensitive. They develop within the nucleus of the host cell and may pass quietly into the cytoplasm and leave the cell without necessarily destroying it. An acidophilic inclusion body surrounded by a halo (Cowdry type A) is characteristically left in the nucleus as a memorial to viral replication. Many viruses in the group show a marked tendency to latency and may become active whenever host immunity is impaired.

Varicella (chickenpox)

Varicella is a highly infectious disease mainly affecting young children, although no age group is exempt. Infection is usually acquired by direct contact with a case during the first few days of illness, when virus is being shed from the respiratory mucosa and skin. The virus is probably transmitted by the airborne route and enters through the respiratory passages. The incubation period varies but commonly lies between 15 and 18 days. In children varicella is generally mild and complications are rare; in adults the illness tends to be more severe with a higher incidence of complications.

The viruses causing chickenpox and herpes zoster appear to be identical and have been designated *Herpesvirus varicellae/zoster.*

Virology and pathology

213 Electron micrograph of *Herpesvirus varicellae/zoster*. On electron microscopy the viruses of varicella, herpes zoster, and herpes simplex are identical. The fully mature particle in the vesicular fluid measures about 150–200 nm in diameter. There is an electron-dense inner core of DNA enclosed by a shell or capsid. This capsid has an icosahedral structure with an axial symmetry of 5:3:2, and consists of 162 capsomeres, which appear as hollow cylinders with a polygonal cross-section. The outer membrane of the virus is derived from the nuclear membrane of the host cell. Herpesviruses are easily distinguished from poxvirus by electron microscopy.

214 *Herpesvirus varicellae/zoster* in human amnion cells. Chickenpox virus does not grow on the chorioallantosis of chick embryos, but can be propagated in a variety of primary cultures of human tissues and in some cultures of monkey tissues. In human amnion culture focal lesions appear in the cell sheet and spread slowly outwards as contagious cells become infected. Typical intranuclear inclusion bodies are found in the degenerate cells. The supernatant fluid remains free from virus. Chickenpox virus grows readily in human thyroid cells and may be harvested from the supernatant fluid for neutralisation tests. (Arrow = cell with intranuclear inclusion.)

215 Giant cell in human amnion cell culture. Multinucleated giant cells are a characteristic feature in human tissues or in cultures of cells infected with chickenpox virus. The nuclei of these cells contain typical eosinophilic type A inclusions. (Arrow = nucleus with inclusion.)

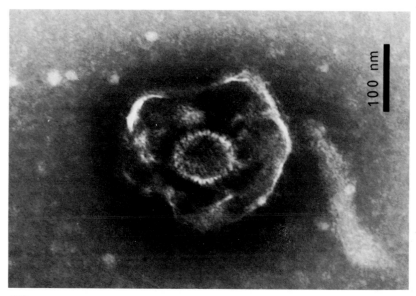

213

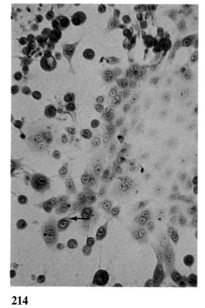

214

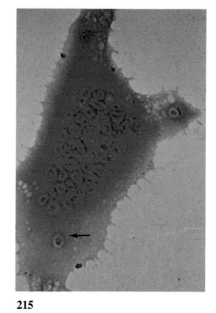

215

185

216 Histology of early chickenpox vesicle. The vesicles of varicella, zoster and herpes simplex cannot be distinguished from each other histologically, but may be differentiated from those of poxvirus infections and vaccinia by the presence of multinucleated giant cells.

Vesicles form within the epidermis as a result of cellular degeneration accompanied by intracellular oedema. At first the fluid collects in small pockets, but these eventually merge to form the mature vesicle.

Two types of degeneration are found – 'ballooning' and reticular. 'Ballooning' is peculiar to virus infections but reticular degeneration is also seen in some forms of dermatitis. In 'ballooning' degeneration the epidermal cells swell, lose their intercellular prickles, and become separated from each other. The cytoplasm is intensely eosinophilic. In reticular degeneration the cells swell but remain clear; some may eventually rupture. (A = intra-epidermal vesicle, B = multinucleated giant cell.)

217 Mature vesicle. The small foci seen in **216** have now coalesced to form a large vesicle. There is little cellular reaction in the dermis and the epithelial cells usually survive intact, so scarring seldom follows. An occasional polymorphonuclear cell may be present in the vesicular fluid. (A = intra-epidermal vesicle, B = dermis.)

Clinical features

218 Distribution of rash. A prodromal illness seldom occurs in children, but occasionally the exanthem in adults may be preceded by fever, headache, and sore throat.

Skin lesions are seen first on the body and inner aspects of the thighs but spread quickly to the face, scalp, and proximal parts of the limbs. The distribution of the rash used to be supremely important in differentiating varicella from variola. The rash in chickenpox is heaviest on the trunk and diminishes in intensity towards the periphery. It is prominent on flexor surfaces and extends into the hollows of the body.

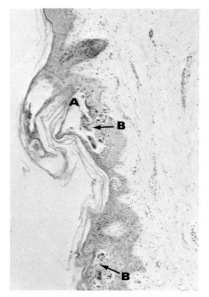

216

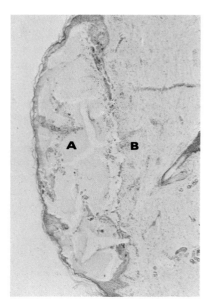

217

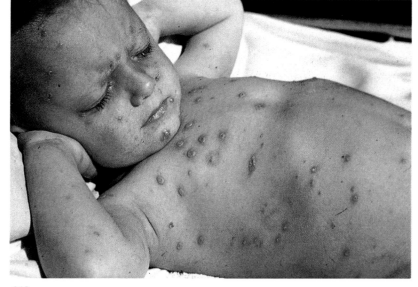

218

219 Chickenpox rash on dark skin. Detection of a chickenpox rash on heavily pigmented skin is easy: although the individual lesions may appear slightly different, the rash conforms to the rule of centripetal distribution. In this illustration the spots are dense on the arm but gradually diminish on the forearm to become scanty on the hand.

220 Pleomorphic rash. The rash evolves very rapidly through the stages of macule, papule, vesicle, pustule, and crust. The first two stages are seldom seen, and the rash usually reaches the vesicular stage before it is discovered. Many lesions abort without undergoing full development.

In chickenpox the lesions emerge in crops at irregular intervals up to a week. As a result, the rash has a pleomorphic character with spots at different stages of development. Pruritus may be very troublesome during the first few days.

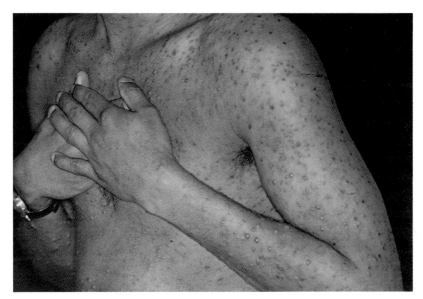

219

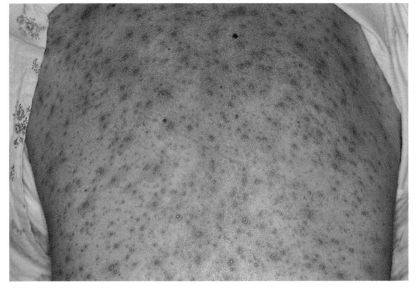

220

221 Close-up of rash on dark skin. In dark-skinned patients it is very common to find a petechial element in the rash and bleeding into the vesicles. The prognosis is not affected by these skin haemorrhages.

222 Close-up of lesions on light skin. Skin lesions vary greatly in size and shape. Fully developed vesicles and pustules are often oval but may be round or totally irregular. The long axis of the oval lesion tends to follow the natural creases of the skin. Many lesions heal at an early stage. Skin haemorrhages are rare in Caucasian patients.

The chickenpox vesicle is unilocular and lies on the surface of the skin like a drop of water. When mature it is often surrounded by an erythematous ring or areola. After 2 or 3 days the vesicular fluid becomes cloudy, and a pustule forms with crenated edges.

223 Scarring. Most chickenpox lesions are very superficial, and damaged epidermis is quickly restored, leaving the skin unblemished. Occasionally the damage extends more deeply into the skin, and unsightly scarring results.

224 Close-up of scar. A pitted or foveated scar is the only clinical evidence that a patient has previously had chickenpox. Similar scars may be produced by vaccination against smallpox or by BCG immunisation.

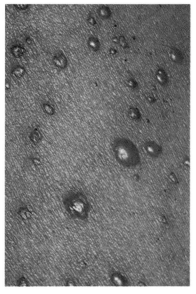

221

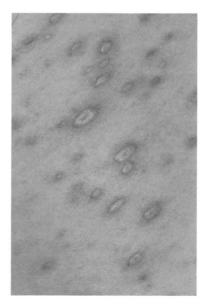

222

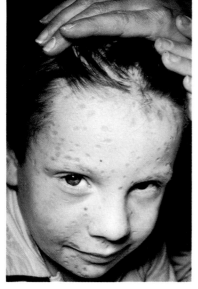

223

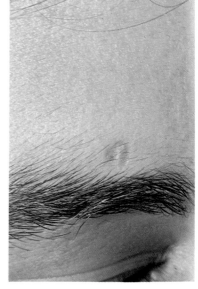

224

225 Petechiae on the palate. Fine haemorrhages may be found on the palate in varicella, as in many other infections. A vesicle is beginning to form on the palate above the left tonsil.

226 Vesicles on the palate. During the first day or two the throat may be painful and inflamed, but no focal lesions are seen. Vesicles may later erupt on the palate and pharynx adding to the discomfort. The thin roof of the vesicle usually ruptures and leaves a shallow ulcer, which heals without scarring.

227 Vesicles on the tongue. Vesicles may be found on the mucosa of the mouth and respiratory tract. On the tongue vesicles have a flat top and heal without forming a crust.

228 Vesicle on the conjunctiva. Vesicles may be found on the conjunctiva, where they pursue a benign course and heal without scarring.

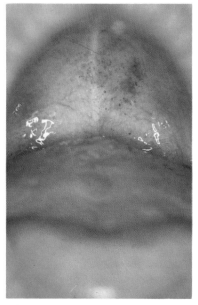

225

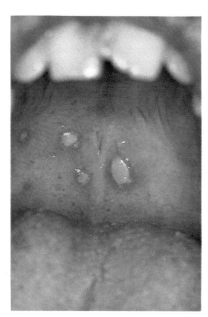

226

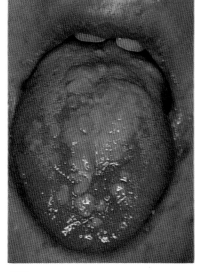

227

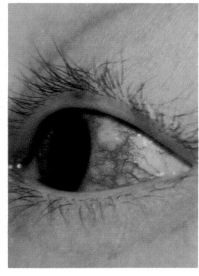

228

Complications

229   Varicella and bullous impetigo. Secondary infection of chickenpox lesions with *Staphylococcus aureus* may give rise to bullous impetigo, with widespread infection of the surface of the skin.

230   Gangrene of the skin. Invasion of the deeper layers of the skin and subcutaneous tissues by a virulent staphylococcus may result in cellulitis with gangrene and deep ulceration.

Septicaemia may develop, with or without evidence of local sepsis, and blood cultures should be performed whenever a patient is unusually ill, or the fever unduly prolonged.

231   Varicella and 'surgical' scarlet fever – rash. Local infection of a chickenpox lesion by a haemolytic streptococcus in a patient susceptible to erythrogenic toxin may result in an attack of scarlet fever. The infected lesions can be identified by the surrounding inflammation. Toxin is absorbed from the skin and produces the generalised punctate erythema of scarlet fever.

232   Varicella and 'surgical' scarlet fever – tongue. Although the streptococcus is growing in the skin and not in the throat, the patient develops a typical enanthem with a white strawberry tongue (see **19**).

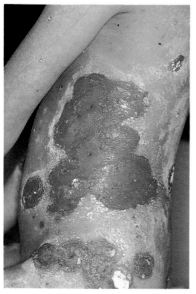

229

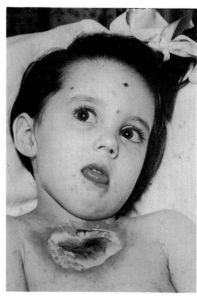

230

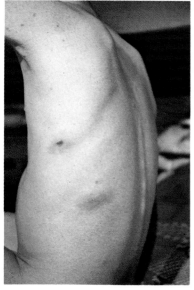

231

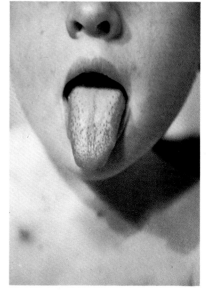

232

233 Chest radiograph of a child with staphylococcal pyopneumothorax.
Pneumonia complicating chickenpox in children is usually caused by secondary
bacterial invasion from the upper respiratory passages, and is predominantly
staphylococcal. Abscesses may form in the lungs.

This child's chest radiograph shows gross displacement of the mediastinum
caused by pyopneumothorax, which resulted from rupture of a subpleural
abscess. Each time the child coughed more air was forced into the pleural cavity
through the pulmonary fistula, and continuous suction was necessary to reduce
the pressure. Pus aspirated from the chest gave a heavy growth of *Staph. aureus*.

234 Chickenpox pneumonia. Chest radiograph – first week. Chickenpox
viral pneumonia is found typically in adult patients and only very exceptionally
in children. The condition varies greatly in severity: at one extreme it is so mild
that it can be detected only by routine radiography; at the other it presents as a
catastrophic illness with severe dyspnoea, cyanosis, haemoptysis, and prostration, terminating fatally within 24–48 hours.

In a typical case the lungs are affected within 2–5 days from the onset of the
rash. During the first week of the illness the characteristic findings are those of
acute inflammatory pulmonary oedema. Dyspnoea and cyanosis are prominent.
Radiographic examination of the chest at this stage shows widespread soft nodular opacities throughout both lungs, but less noticeable at the apices.

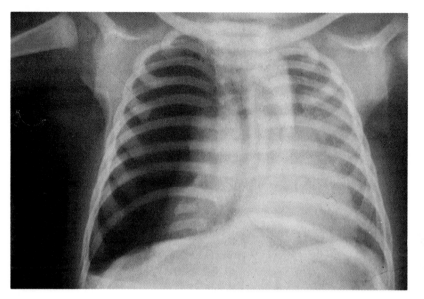

233

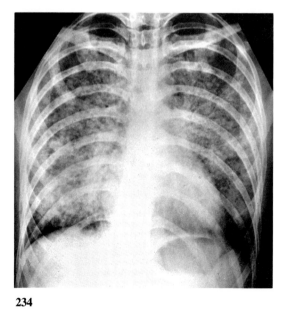

234

235 Chickenpox pneumonia. Chest radiograph – second week. Mortality is high in pregnant women and in patients with disturbed immunity, who commonly die from respiratory failure during the first week. During the second week the pulmonary oedema abates and the patient begins to improve. The cough lessens, and the abnormal chest signs disappear. Towards the end of the second week the chest radiograph shows changes as the soft nodular shadowing resolves, leaving a prominent reticular pattern.

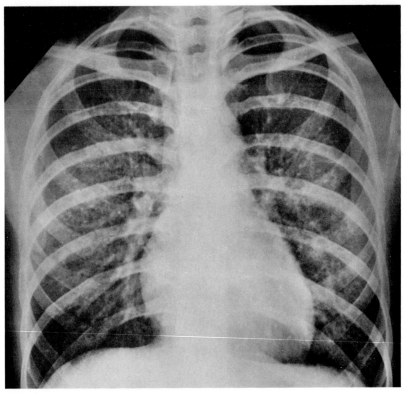

235

236 Chickenpox pneumonia. Chest radiograph – miliary calcification.
After 2 weeks the patient emerges from the acute stage to face a prolonged period of convalescence. Breathlessness on slight exertion may persist for several
weeks or months, but eventually subsides, and full health is restored. In most
patients the coarse reticular pattern gradually fades, although the chest radiograph may reveal abnormalities for many months. Patients found on routine
examination to have miliary calcification of the lungs often give a history of
severe chickenpox in adult life, and it is believed that calcium salts are deposited
in the necrotic foci that are a typical feature of chickenpox penumonia. Similar
appearances may be found as a result of histoplasmosis or miliary tuberculosis.

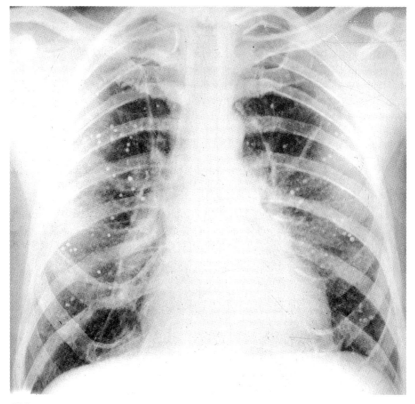

236

237 Chickenpox pneumonia – histology of lung. In fatal cases of chickenpox pneumonia the lungs are grossly oedematous, and there are extensive haemorrhages. Histological examination shows widely disseminated interstitial pneumonia with patchy haemorrhagic consolidation.

The illustration shows a 3mm focus of fibrinoid necrosis surrounded by a zone of septal oedema and haemorrhage.

238 Chickenpox pneumonia – alveolar exudate. The alveoli are filled with a protein-rich fluid containing red cells and mononuclear cells. To the left of centre may be seen a degenerate mononuclear cell with a typical intranuclear inclusion. The nuclear membrane is clearly visible, but the cytoplasm is faintly stained. (Arrow = nuclear membrane with inclusion body.)

239 Haemorrhagic chickenpox. Widespread, and sometimes fatal, bleeding into the skin and mucous membranes may be precipitated by a number of infections, including chickenpox. The extent of the haemorrhages is not necessarily related to the severity of the original illness. In haemorrhagic chickenpox the platelet count is very low, the prothrombin time prolonged, and there may be other evidence of excessive consumption of clotting factors. Intravascular coagulation and endothelial damage by the virus may both contribute to the patient's death. Extensive haemorrhages into the skin or mucous membranes may be accompanied by alarming epistaxis, haematemesis, or haematuria.

240 Concurrent varicella and measles. The importance of the interference phenomenon varies with different virus infections. Sometimes infection with one virus may completely prevent invasion by another. This applies particularly to closely related viruses, such as members of the enterovirus group, but seldom occurs when viruses have notably different characteristics.

In the illustration a chickenpox rash is emerging on the upper limb of a child with a florid measles rash.

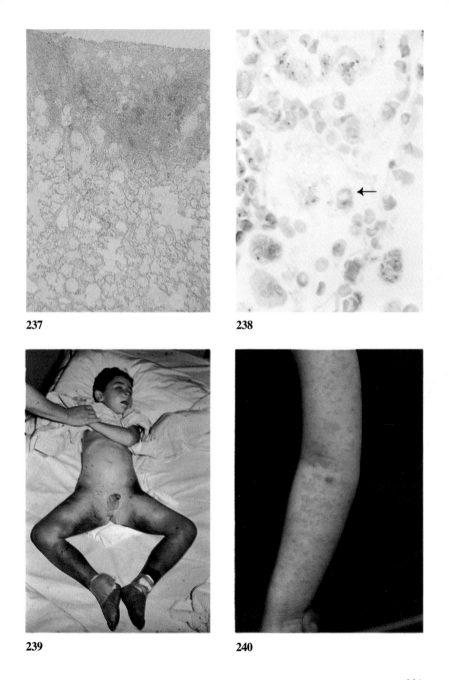

237

238

239

240

Varicella in disturbed immunity

241 Varicella and disturbed immunity. Patients with underlying disease affecting immunity are especially vulnerable to chickenpox, which may follow an exceptionally severe or prolonged course and may terminate in death.

The illustration shows a patient with Hodgkin's disease who contracted chickenpox from her child. Although the rash was not particularly dense, the individual lesions were unusually large and the general disturbance severe. Jaundice developed and 'cropping' continued until the patient died 3 or 4 weeks after the onset of her illness.

242 Close-up of lesions in chickenpox associated with disturbed immunity. The large size of the lesions is striking. The pustular fluid was sterile on culture for bacteria.

Patients who have never had chickenpox and who have defective immunity as a result of disease of the reticuloendothelial system or immunosuppressive treatment, are in grave danger from chickenpox and should not be exposed to this disease or to herpes zoster. If a patient has been inadvertently exposed, passive immunisation with varicella/zoster immunoglobulin should be considered.

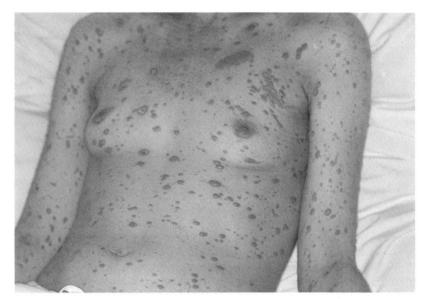

241

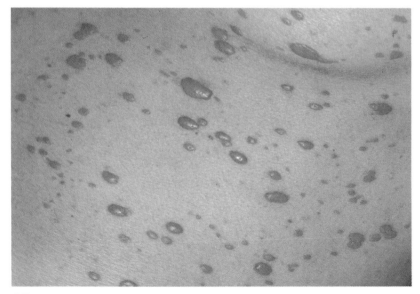

242

Herpes zoster (shingles)

Pathology

243 Histology of the dorsal root ganglion. Herpes zoster is thought to be caused by reactivation of varicella virus lying dormant in cells of a dorsal root ganglion. In the early stages there is an acute inflammatory reaction in the ganglion, or its equivalent in the cranial nerves, which extends into the dorsal root and involves the meninges and spinal cord. Mononuclear cells are conspicuous, but there is a notable absence of polymorphonuclear cells. (A = undegenerate neurones, B = degenerate neurones, C = mononuclear cells.)

244 Histology of peripheral nerve. Virus spreads from the dorsal root ganglion cells along the sensory nerve fibres to the skin, where it enters the epithelial cells. At this stage virus particles may be found in the nuclei and cytoplasm of ganglion cells, in the cytoplasm of perineural cells, in the nuclei and cytoplasm of Schwann cells, and in the nuclei and cytoplasm of cells in the epidermis.

The illustration shows a section of frontal nerve from a patient with trigeminal herpes, who died 4 days after the onset of the rash. Staining by fluorescent antibody demonstrates viral antigen in two nerve fibre bundles with heavy concentration in the perineurium.

245 Histology of vesicle. The vesicles of herpes zoster and varicella are identical. The vesicle forms in the epidermis as a result of degeneration of the cells, which become swollen and separated, and some rupture. Intercellular oedema is marked and giant cells are a prominent feature. Severe inflammatory reaction in the corium may be followed by scarring.

In this section inflammatory reaction is slight, but many bizarre cells are present. (A = intraepidermal vesicle, B = multinucleated giant cell, C = dermis.)

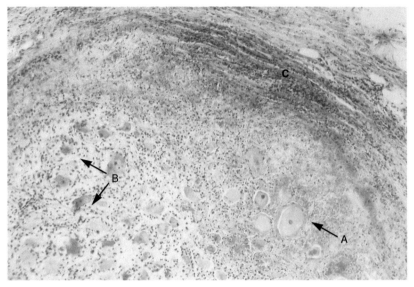

243

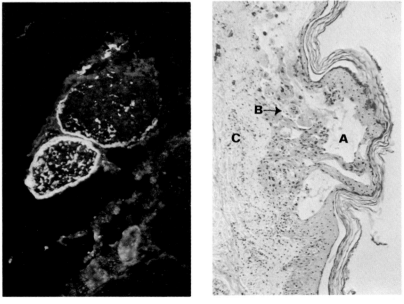

244

245

246 Effect of nerve damage on distribution of the rash. A patient with hypoaesthesia, a result of section of a cutaneous nerve during a herniotomy 15 months previously, developed an attack of herpes zoster involving the same dermatome. Virus spread readily into the skin where sensation was normal, but round the scar, where the nerve supply had been interrupted, the skin was spared. This would be expected if the virus in herpes zoster gains access to the epidermis along nerve pathways.

Clinical features

247 Evolution of rash – erythema. An attack of herpes zoster begins with pain and hyperaesthesia in the distribution of one or two adjacent sensory nerve roots. Within a few days a rash appears in the same area. At first the skin has a deep red flush, but clusters of vesicles soon emerge. The rash is strictly confined by the midline, but oedema may spread extensively wherever subcutaneous tissues are lax.

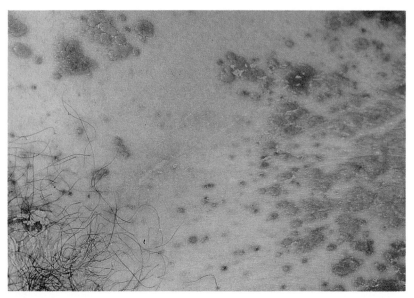

246

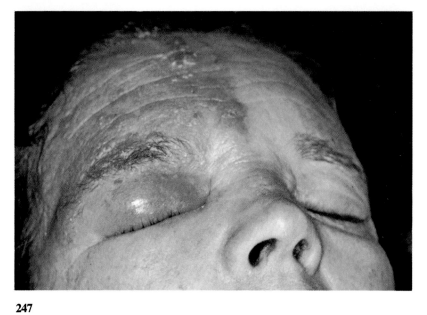

247

248 Evolution of rash – vesicles. The severity of the illness and extent of the rash are extremely variable. Fresh crops of vesicles continue to emerge for several days and may coalesce to form bullae, some of which may be haemorrhagic.

249 Evolution of rash – pustules. After a week or so the vesicles begin to dry up and form scabs but some may go through an intermediate pustular stage. These are usually sterile on bacterial culture.

250 Evolution of rash – crusts. If the rash is heavy, and especially if there is damage to the underlying corium, a thick plate of scabs may form which takes several weeks to separate. Any attempt at forcible removal merely results in the formation of fresh scabs and further harm to the skin. With a rash of average severity the scabs have usually been shed within 2 or 3 weeks.

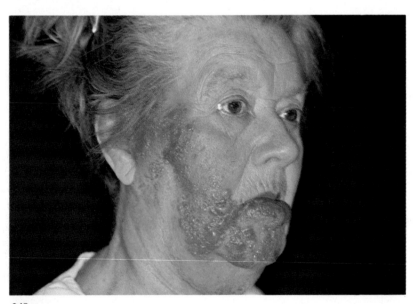

248

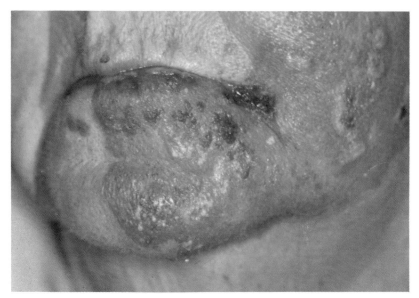

249

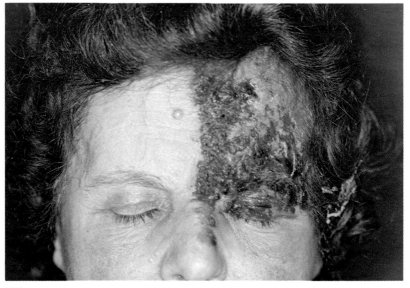

250

251 Evolution of rash ulcers. In most attacks the skin will heal without scars. Should the crusts separate and produce deep ulceration then scarring is inevitable. Heavy pigmentation may persist in the damaged area for many months.

252 Close-up of vesicles. The vesicles develop in clusters on an erythematous base.

253 Close-up of pustules. At a later stage the fluid in the blisters becomes turbid, and pustules are formed. This is not due to secondary bacterial invasion but to the activity of the virus itself. Adjacent lesions tend to run into each other, and already a central crust is appearing. Haemorrhage is common in severe attacks and produces bluish discoloration.

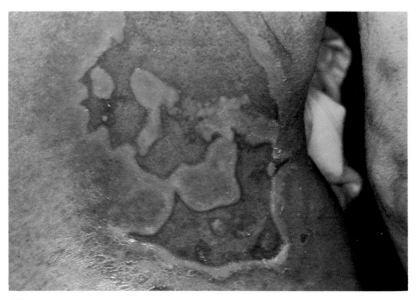

251

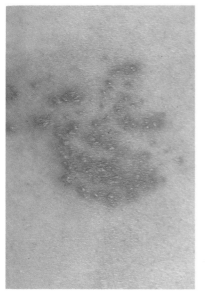

252

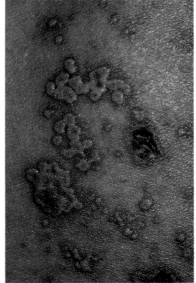

253

254 Distribution – cervical. The rash has sharply defined borders confined to the areas of skin supplied by cervical roots 4 and 5. This peculiar segmental distribution is a very helpful feature making it possible to distinguish herpes zoster from other similar rashes, particularly erysipelas (see **22**). Herpes simplex may simulate zoster, but pain is less troublesome, and the rash seldom conforms to a complete segmental distribution (see **293**).

255 Distribution – thoracic. Thoracic segments are affected in over 50% of patients with zoster. The rash is distributed in a band around the trunk. The term zoster is derived from the Greek (meaning belt), and shingles from the Low Latin equivalent.

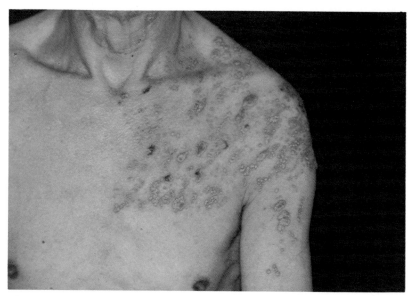

254

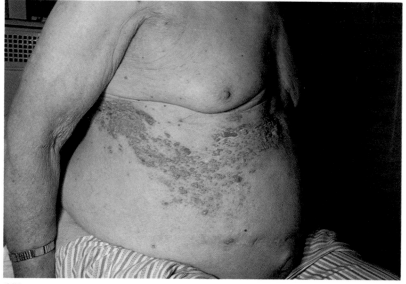

255

256 Distribution – thoracic. The rash seldom covers the entire area of skin in a dermatome. Lesions are grouped in clusters and generally form an unmistakable pattern. The diagnosis may be difficult when the eruption consists of a single cluster, but a history of pain preceding the spots provides a helpful clue. In doubtful cases diagnosis can be established by demonstrating a rising antibody concentration in paired sera.

257 Herpes zoster with a generalised rash. If patients with herpes zoster are examined carefully, at least half will be found to have a sparse chickenpox rash. This emerges after the zoster, and the spots often abort at an early stage of development.

Moderate or heavy generalised varicella eruptions occur in 2–4% of cases, and are common when there is an underlying disturbance of immunity.

The standard sequence of events is reactivation of virus in the dorsal root ganglion, with spread of virus along the sensory nerves to the skin segment, followed by dissemination into the blood stream resulting in a generalised rash.

258 Herpes zoster in a child. Herpes zoster is predominantly a disease of the middle-aged and elderly: less than 5% of attacks occur in children below the age of 10 years. When zoster develops in very young children there is frequently a history of an attack of chickenpox in the mother during pregnancy. Postherpetic neuralgia is seldom a problem in children.

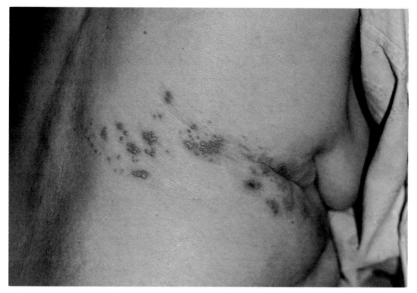

256

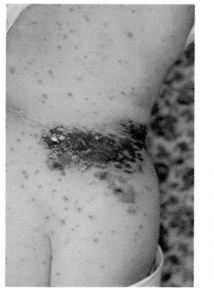

257

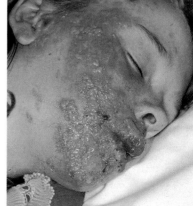

258

259 Herpes zoster of the palate. When an appropriate ganglion is affected lesions may be found on mucous membranes. Herpes zoster of the second division of the fifth cranial nerve affects the palate as well as the skin over the maxilla.

Complications

260 Conjunctivitis. Conjunctivitis may persist for several weeks after an attack of ophthalmic herpes, especially in the elderly, and may be associated with keratitis or iridocyclitis.

261 Corneal ulceration. During convalescence, after an attack of ophthalmic herpes, minor trauma to the anaesthetised cornea may abrade the surface and result in troublesome ulceration. Continual dabbing at the painful watering eye by an elderly confused patient may produce a penetrating ulcer that could perforate the anterior chamber. In these circumstances tarsorrhaphy may be required to protect the eye until the ulcer heals.

262 Chemosis. Unilateral ophthalmic herpes may be accompanied by oedema of the eyelids on both sides of the face and by striking oedema of the conjunctiva on the affected side (chemosis). When the eyelids are opened, the oedematous conjunctiva protrudes as a yellow gelatinous bag. The condition is not serious and resolves quickly.

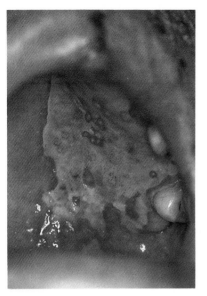

259

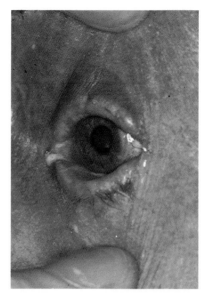

260

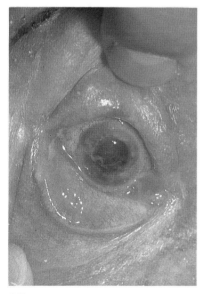

261

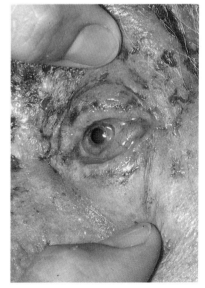

262

263 Iridocyclitis. The first division of the trigeminal nerve supplies the skin of the forehead and also the iris and ciliary body. A heavy rash on the side of the nose indicates that the nasociliary branch is severely affected, and iridocyclitis a strong probability.

The patient usually has difficulty in opening the oedematous eyelids so may not complain of defective vision. On examination the cornea is hazy and the pupil small. The reaction of the pupil is impaired, and the colour of the iris is altered. When the pupil is dilated by a mydriatic the outline may be irregular as a result of adhesions between the iris and cornea.

264 Streptococcal impetigo. If herpetic lesions are kept dry, secondary bacterial infection is seldom a problem. Superimposed streptococcal infection may cause impetigo or erysipelas.

265 Secondary staphylococcal infection. A combination of zoster with a virulent staphylococcal infection may result in extensive damage to the corium and ugly scarring.

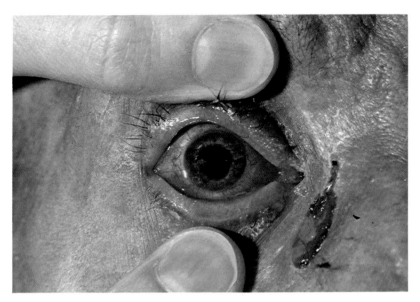

263

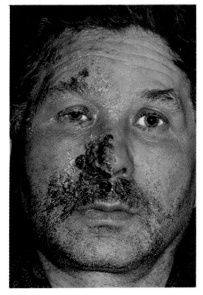

264

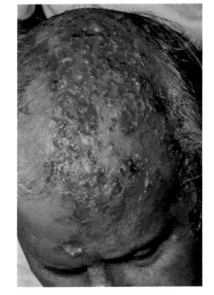

265

266 Herpes zoster with ophthalmoplegia. Spread of virus to lower motor neurone cells is not uncommon, and minor degrees of weakness are easily overlooked.

This patient had an attack of zoster involving the ophthalmic division of the fifth nerve complicated by ophthalmoplegia. He has ptosis and is unable to move his right eye. The conjunctiva is severely congested.

267 Facial paralysis complicating herpes zoster. Facial paralysis may follow herpes zoster of the trigeminal nerve, the geniculate ganglion of the seventh, or the second and third cervical roots. The exact pathways traversed by the virus are unknown.

This patient had zoster of the fifth cranial nerve, which resulted in facial weakness of lower motor neurone type and severe postherpetic neuralgia.

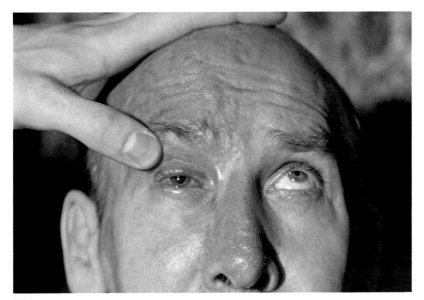

266

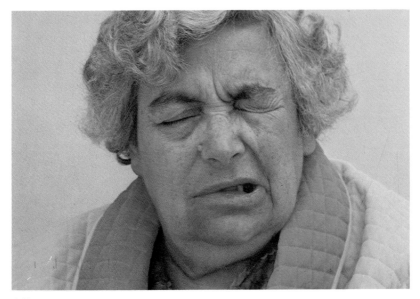

267

268   Geniculate herpes. Zoster of the geniculate ganglion of the seventh cranial nerve produces a crop of vesicles on the pinna and gives rise to facial paralysis accompanied by loss of taste over the anterior two-thirds of the tongue. Deafness may occur. The prognosis depends on the initial severity of the weakness.

269   Herpes zoster of C2 and C3 with facial paralysis. The patient has widespread zoster of the right side of her neck complicated by facial paralysis and deafness. She is unable to close her right eye, and her mouth is drawn over to the left. A year later the paralysis showed no improvement.

270   Herpes zoster of C4 and C5 with paralysis. During an attack of zoster affecting the fourth and fifth cervical roots, this elderly patient complained of 'rheumatism' in her right shoulder. Examination revealed that the stiffness was caused by weakness of the shoulder muscles. In attempting to abduct her arm the patient compensated for the deltoid paralysis by raising her shoulder and rotating her scapula.

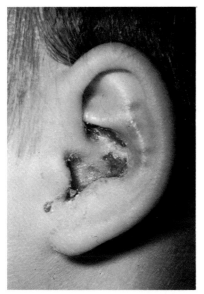

268

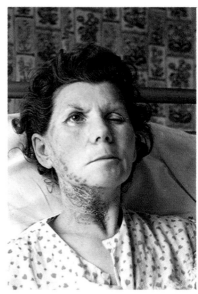

269

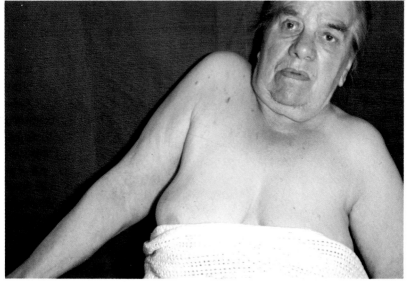

270

271 Diaphragmatic paralysis in herpes zoster. Herpes zoster of C4 may occasionally be complicated by diaphragmatic paralysis. On routine radiographic examination during convalescence from an attack of herpes zoster the diaphragm was found to be markedly raised on the left side.

272 and 273   Horner's syndrome. The autonomic nervous system may also be affected by herpes zoster. This patient, with zoster of T2, developed Horner's syndrome on the affected side. Enophthalmos and a small pupil persisted for a few weeks, then cleared.

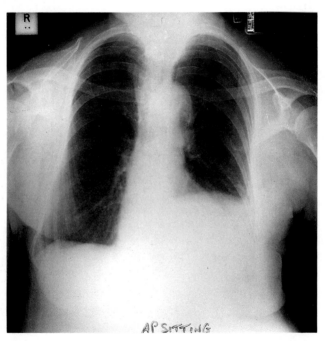

271

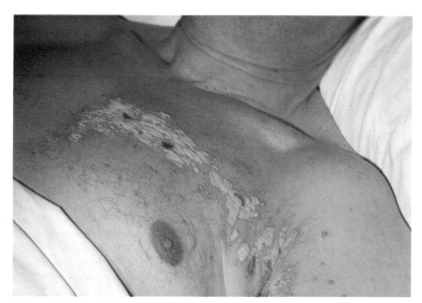

272

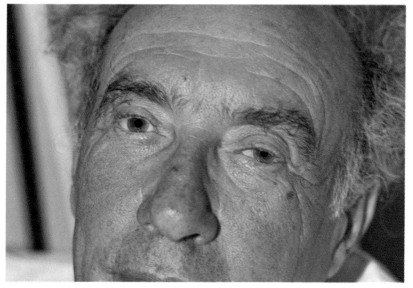

273

Herpes zoster and disturbed immunity

274 Herpes zoster and leukaemia. An attack of herpes zoster may be precipitated by any condition that depresses immunity and allows the latent virus to emerge. All patients with zoster should be examined carefully for enlarged lymph nodes, splenomegaly, or hepatomegaly. The presence of undiagnosed lymphatic leukaemia may be signposted by an attack of shingles.

275 Herpes zoster and Hodgkin's disease. About 8% of patients admitted to hospital with zoster are found to have an underlying disease such as leukaemia, Hodgkin's disease, or carcinomatosis. Attacks may also be precipitated by immunosuppressive treatment. In such patients the skin lesions are often haemorrhagic and necrotic. The general disturbance is severe, and many patients die.

276 Herpes zoster and carcinomatosis. Metastases from surgically treated breast cancer were discovered when the patient developed a severe attack of herpes zoster and a heavy chickenpox rash. Many of the skin lesions are necrotic and the patient is jaundiced. The liver is enlarged and the abdomen distended by ascites. Radiographic examination of the chest showed secondary deposits in the lungs.

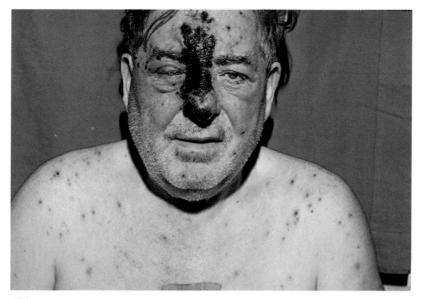

274

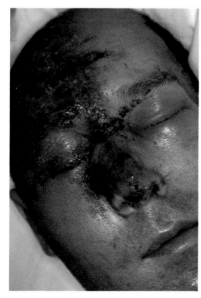

275

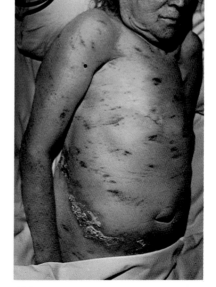

276

Herpes simplex infections

Primary infection with herpes simplex virus usually occurs in early childhood but may be deferred until adult life. In most children the reaction to the initial invasion is trivial, with a few sores around the mouth, but a few develop acute gingivostomatitis and may be extremely ill. Subclinical infections are not uncommon. Once acquired, the virus may remain dormant for many years in cells of sensory nerve ganglia and has been detected in a high proportion of ganglia removed immediately after death.

Recurrent attacks are common and generally infect the skin around the mouth, although other sites may be affected. Herpes simplex virus is also responsible for infections of the central nervous system, eye, and genital tract; it is suspected to be an aetiological factor in squamous carcinoma of the lip and in carcinoma of the cervix of the uterus. Patients with eczema are especially susceptible to the virus and may succumb to generalised infection.

Herpes simplex virus of humans is one of a large group of similar viruses naturally infecting many mammals and birds. Of these, only B virus of monkeys is known to cause human disease. Herpes simplex virus can be separated into two types, according to antigenic differences and biological characteristics. A small number of strains do not fall readily into either group.

Virology

277 Herpes simplex virus type 1 on chorioallantoic membrane. Type 1 viruses are usually isolated from the mouth or throat, from skin lesions, or from the brain of adults with encephalitis.

All human strains of the virus grow readily on chick embryo. Lesions appear on the chorioallantois within 24–28 hours after inoculation, and reach their maximum size in 3–4 days. The pocks produced by type 1 virus are smaller (less than 0.5 mm diameter) but more numerous than those produced by type 2. They are also more superficial.

278 Herpes simplex virus type 2 on chorioallantoic membrane. Type 2 viruses are usually isolated from the genital tract but may be recovered from brain and other organs in neonatal infection.

Fewer lesions are produced on chorioallantoic membrane by type 2 viruses but the lesions are large (more than 1 mm in diameter), and more deeply seated.

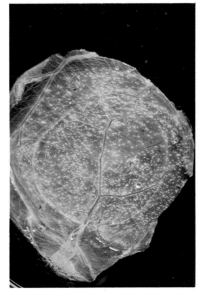 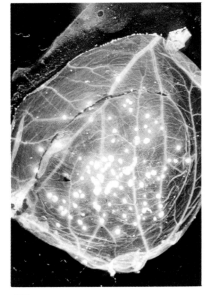

277 278

279   Normal monkey kidney cell culture.

280   Herpes simplex virus in monkey kidney cells. Chick embryo is no longer used for primary isolation of herpes simplex virus but is still used for confirming the type. Isolation of the virus is accomplished more easily in tissue cultures of primary rabbit kidney or primary human amnion cells, although many other cells are suitable. The growth of the virus can be recognised by cytopathogenic changes, which appear within 24–48 hours. These vary with the type of virus and the nature of the host cells. A lytic effect is produced in amnion cells and multinucleated giant cells may be found in HeLa cell cultures. In monkey kidney cell culture the infected cells degenerate and become rounded.

Clinical syndromes

281   Disseminated herpes infection in a neonate. Focal necrosis of liver. Spread of infection from the mother's genital tract at birth, or from an attendant may result in severe generalised infection culminating in death. Evidence of infection usually appears 4–5 days after birth. Local lesions may be found on the surface of the body but these are quickly overshadowed by the catastrophic general disturbance.

Foci of miliary necrosis are found in many organs and are particularly prominent in the liver. The condition may be mistaken for miliary tuberculosis. (Arrows = necrotic foci.)

282   Acute disseminated herpes – histology of the liver. Intranuclear inclusion bodies are found in cells adjacent to areas of necrosis. When fully developed the inclusion is eosinophilic and Feulgen-negative. An unstained halo separates the inclusion from the nuclear membrane.

Around the edge of the lesion some of the cells show evidence of impending necrosis. These cells may be identified by the pyknotic nuclei.

Herpes simplex virus type 2 is found in 80% of neonates with disseminated infection. (A = intranuclear inclusion, B = pyknotic nucleus.)

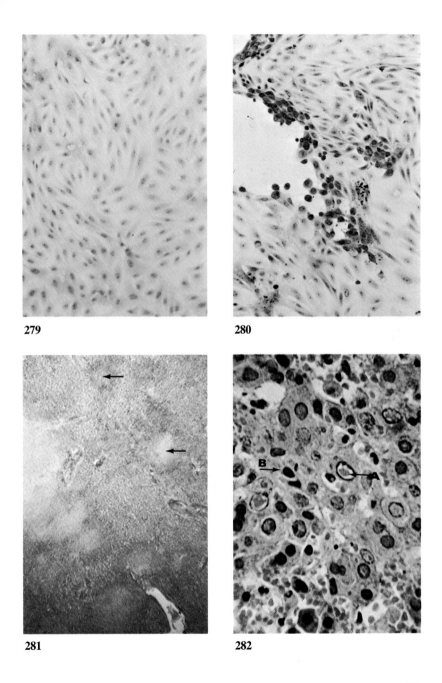

279

280

281

282

283   Herpetic encephalitis – section of the brain. Infection of the central nervous system is more common than was previously thought. It may manifest as a meningo-encephalitis or encephalitis, generally associated with type 1 virus, or as aseptic meningitis, myelitis or radiculitis, generally associated with type 2 virus.

At autopsy there is intense engorgement of the brain and meninges with perivascular cuffing around the vessels in the cortex and subcortical white matter. The brain tissue is infiltrated with lymphocytes, plasma cells, and large mononuclear cells. Intranuclear inclusion bodies are found mainly in glial cells, but are also present in nerve cells.

Older children and adults may develop a localised form of encephalitis, mainly affecting the temporal lobe, which presents clinically as a space-occupying lesion. Necrosis is a striking feature of this localised form.

The section of brain shows perivascular cuffing with lymphocytes, plasma cells, and mononuclear cells. There are no polymorphonuclear cells or inclusions.

284   Neurones infected with herpes simplex virus. Fluorescent antibody staining shows viral antigens in nerve cells from a fatal case of herpetic encephalitis.

285   Acute disseminated herpes in an older child. Fatal dissemination of the virus may occur in older children suffering from malnutrition. The changes in the tissues are similar to those found in neonatal infection. Type 1 virus is usually responsible.

This section of liver from an African child has been stained by fluorescent-antibody technique, which indicates the presence of viral antigen along the portal tract.

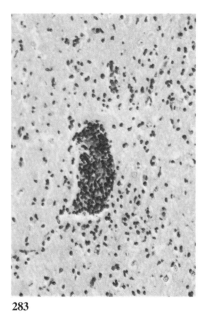

283

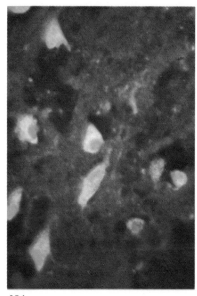

284

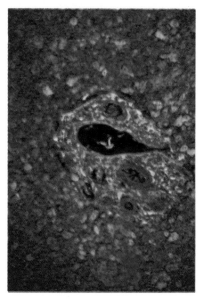

285

286 Histology of vesicle. At onset of infection cells in the deeper layers of the epidermis proliferate, but degenerative changes soon follow. The affected cells swell, become separated from each other and some eventually rupture. Multinucleated giant cells may form. The underlying dermis is infiltrated by moderate numbers of neutrophil polymorphonuclear cells and lymphocytes.

The section is from hairy skin and shows a superficial vesicle that has destroyed the epidermis. The roof of the vesicle has collapsed and part of it may be seen at each side of the lesion. (A = edges of roof of vesicle, B = dermis, C = hair follicle, D = subcutaneous tissue.)

287 Primary gingivostomatitis in a child. Herpes simplex virus is a very successful parasite and infection is widespread. In most communities about 60% of the population over five to six years old possess antibody against type 1 virus. Subclinical or mild infection is very common in early childhood, but primary infection in young children may occasionally provoke severe gingivostomatitis.

After a short prodromal illness lesions appear in the mouth. These consist of thin-walled vesicles on an erythematous base that soon rupture to form typical shallow ulcers with a serpiginous edge. The gums are particularly inflamed and swollen.

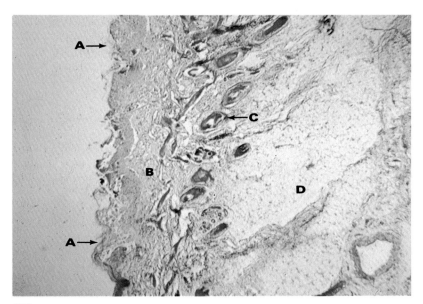

286

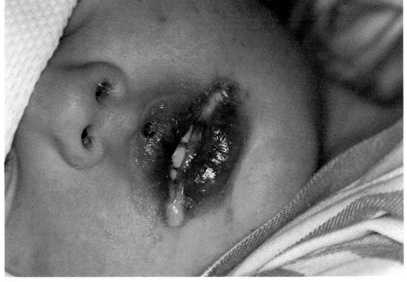

287

288   Stomatitis with secondary lesions on skin. In severe herpetic gingivo-stomatitis the young child becomes acutely ill with a high fever and is reluctant to eat or drink because of pain. Continuous drooling from the infected mouth transfers virus to the skin of the face, neck and chest. After a week the temperature usually returns to normal but another week or two may elapse before the mouth heals.

289   Herpetic gingivostomatitis in an adult. Adult patients with primary infection of the gums may be seen by the dentist rather than the physician. The gums are inflamed and swollen. Initially the vesicles are discrete, but soon run together and burst to form typical serpiginous ulcers. Primary infection in adults is found more commonly in higher socioeconomic groups.

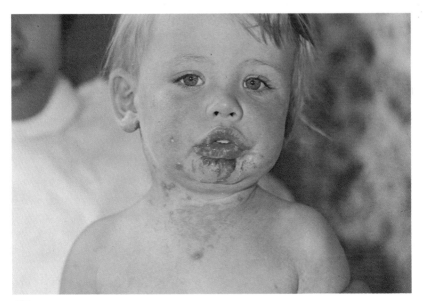

288

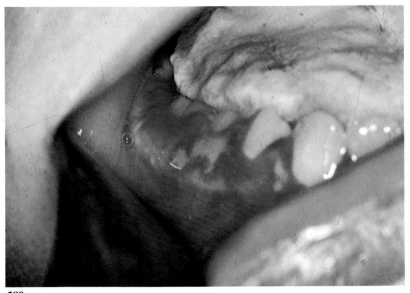

289

237

290 Acute gingivostomatitis in an adult. Primary infection with herpes simplex virus may affect the mouth in adults as well as children. The appearance is similar in both age groups, but the constitutional disturbance is less in adults.

291 Herpetic lesions on the tongue of an adult. The tongue is heavily coated, and small round vesicles are scattered sparsely over the surface. Herpetic stomatitis or glossitis should not be confused with aphthous stomatitis, which is an entirely unrelated condition. Palatal lesions may be mistaken for herpangina (see **423** and **424**).

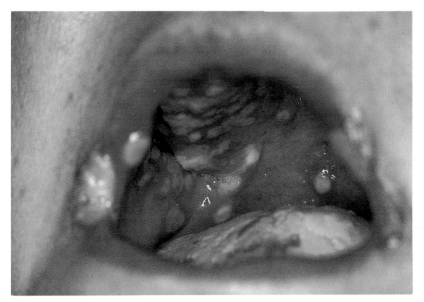

290

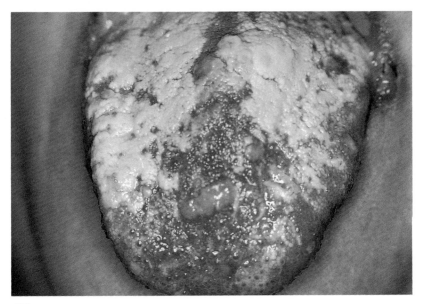

291

292　Primary infection of the skin. Primary infection of the skin is seen more commonly in older children and adults. Spread is by direct contact to any part of the body. Outbreaks amongst wrestlers have been dignified by the title 'herpes gladiatorum'.

293　Herpes simplex mimicking herpes zoster. In some patients herpes simplex infection may closely simulate zoster, and there may even be mild sensory disturbance, but there is less pain and the distribution does not conform to a dermatome. Diagnosis is difficult when herpes zoster affects only part of a root. In these circumstances the shorter prodromal period and the relative absence of pain in simplex infections are points to be considered but, when doubt persists, the diagnosis will be decided by laboratory tests.

This rugby footballer developed a rash on his face after a game and was initially thought to have herpes zoster, but the rapid onset and unusual distribution aroused suspicion, and a diagnosis of primary herpes simplex infection was confirmed by growing the virus and demonstrating a rise in antibody titre.

294　Recurrent infection. Recurrent attacks of herpes simplex infection differ from the primary attack. They occur in older children and adults with high antibody concentrations, and there is no subsequent rise in titre. The attack is often precipitated by a trivial stimulus, but is particularly common in pneumonia, meningitis and malaria. It is highly probable that the virus lies dormant in cells of sensory nerve ganglia and spreads to the skin along cutaneous nerve fibres.

A sensation of tingling or tightness may be felt in the skin for a few hours before the rash appears. Clusters of little vesicles develop rapidly on an erythematous base, usually on the skin round the mouth. The vesicles quickly evolve through pustules to scabs, which separate and heal without leaving scars. Very rarely, a squamous cell carcinoma develops at the site of recurring herpes.

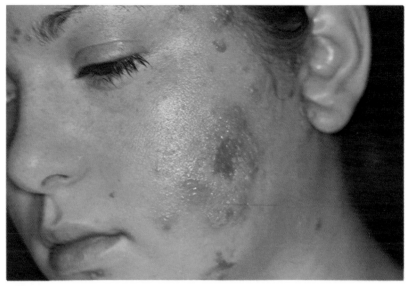

292

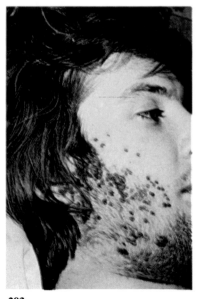

293

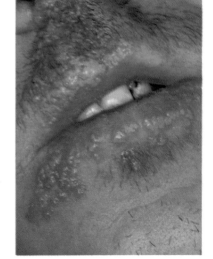

294

295 Herpetic infection of the eye. Herpetic infections of the eye can occur at any age and may be primary or recurrent.

Neonatal eye infections are generally acquired from the mother's genital tract at birth and may be the sole manifestation or else a minor component of disseminated infection.

Primary infection of the eye is most common in children and usually takes the form of unilateral follicular conjunctivitis with pronounced oedema of the conjunctiva and eyelids. Vesicles may be present on the eyelids. Associated infection of the cornea often results in coarse punctate epithelial opacities.

Recurrent herpes is usually seen in adults and may prove exceedingly troublesome. The cornea is predominantly affected, and follicular conjunctivitis is exceptional. Herpetic keratitis varies greatly in severity from superficial dendritic ulceration to inflammation of the deeper layers of the corneal stroma. Topical applications of corticosteroid preparations are dangerous and may convert simple dendritic ulceration into deep amoeboid ulceration with risk of perforation and hypopyon.

The dendritic ulcer in the illustration has been stained with fluorescein.

296 Herpetic whitlow. Nurses and doctors lacking specific antibody are especially susceptible to primary herpetic infection of the fingers. The virus is acquired from patients and readily penetrates the skin through minor cuts and abrasions. Infection is often derived from catheters used for clearing tracheostomy tubes. Herpetic infections of the finger also occur in children and may be secondary to gingivostomatitis.

Herpetic whitlows may take the form of pulpitis or clusters of blisters on the skin. The lesions are painful and there may be a general reaction with fever and headache.

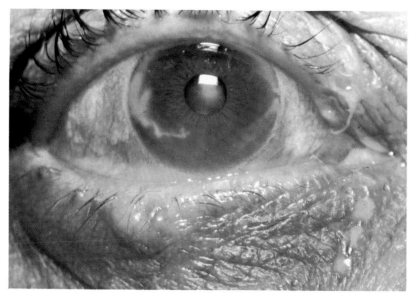

295

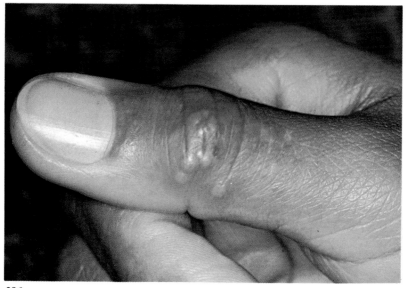

296

297   Eczema herpeticum on the trunk of an adult. Patients with eczema are particularly vulnerable to infection with herpes simplex virus. Infection spreads readily in the eczematous skin, producing crops of small superficial vesicles. These evolve through a pustular stage to form crusts that separate, leaving shallow necrotic ulcers. These eventually heal with a variable degree of scarring.

Systemic invasion may lead to generalised infection and death. Eczema herpeticum is seen most frequently in young children, but occurs occasionally in older children and adults.

298   Eczema herpeticum – close up.

299   Genital herpes – adult man. Genital herpes is usually caused by type 2 virus. Infection is commonly, but not invariably, transmitted by sexual intercourse. The prevalence is much greater in women.

Lesions are detected most often on the prepuce or in the coronal sulcus. They also occur on the shaft of the penis or in the urethra. Latent infection with type 2 virus seems to be common in men but not women. Heaviest infection is found in the vas deferens.

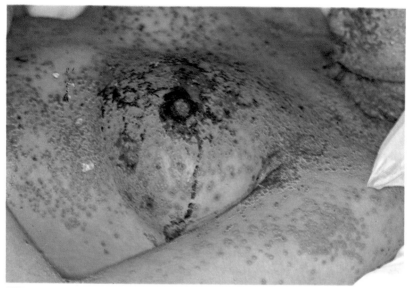

297

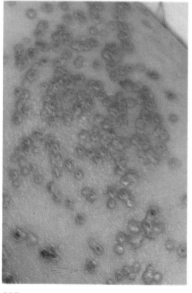

298

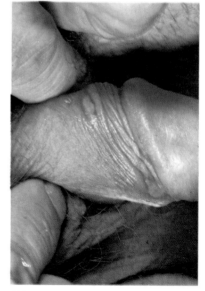

299

300 Genital herpes on the vulva of an adult woman. Herpetic lesions may be found on the vulva, vagina or cervix, and may appear on the perineum or buttocks. Genital herpes in pregnancy may cause overwhelming infection in newborn babies, particularly when they are premature. The very high neonatal mortality makes it necessary to investigate all vesicles or ulcers on the genital tract of pregnant women (see **334**).

301 Genital herpes – cervix of an adult woman. Herpetic cervicitis may result from a primary infection or follow reactivation of latent infection. The genital lesions in women tend to ulcerate rapidly and become covered with exudate. There may be an association between type 2 virus infections and invasive carcinoma of the cervix.

302 Vulvovaginitis in a child. Primary infection of the skin may be found at any site. When the vulva is infected in infants, a diagnosis of 'nappy rash' may be made and the possibility of herpetic infection overlooked.

In herpetic vulvovaginitis the skin is macerated and the labia stuck together by gummy exudate. Vesicles may be inconspicuous.

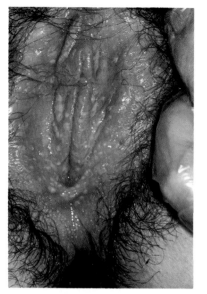

300

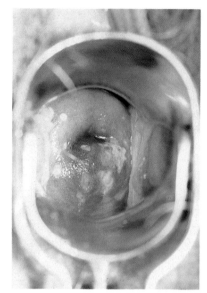

301

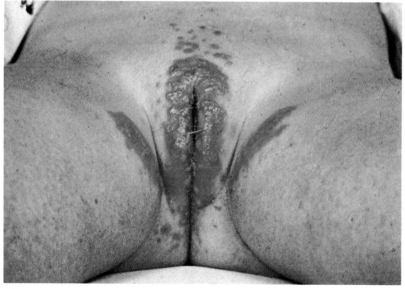

302

Cytomegalovirus infection

Primary infection of the mother during pregnancy may occasionally result in death of the fetus or serious generalised disease closely simulating toxoplasmosis in the newborn. Erythroblastosis, thrombocytopenia with purpura, jaundice, and hepatomegaly are striking features of the illness. More commonly, congenital cytomegalovirus infections follow a benign course, although about 10% of infected children may be mentally retarded.

While postnatal infection in children may cause chronic liver disease, it more frequently remains latent throughout childhood and adolescence. Primary infection in adults may be subclinical, or may present with a variety of syndromes including cytomegalovirus fever, hepatitis, or Paul–Bunnell-negative infectious mononucleosis.

303 Electron micrograph of cytomegalovirus. Cytomegaloviruses are found in humans and various animals. On electron microscopy the virus has the characteristic appearance of a herpesvirus.

304 Cytomegalovirus – section of parotid gland showing inclusion bodies. Cytomegaloviruses have a particular affinity for salivary glands. Large intranuclear inclusion bodies ('owl eye') are found in cells lining the ducts of the salivary glands in 5–25% of babies dying in early infancy. The affected cells are large, with a diameter up to 40 μm. (Arrow indicates a large cell with 'owl eye' inclusion.)

305 Section of kidney showing inclusions. In generalised disease large cells containing inclusions may be found in the lungs, kidneys, pancreas, and other organs. A dilated tubule can be seen in the centre of this renal section. The lining epithelial cells contain large intranuclear inclusions. Enlarged cells with inclusions may be detected in the urine, and virus can be recovered on tissue culture. Infection in children results in prolonged excretion of the virus and therefore it is essential to assess such findings carefully in relation to the clinical picture. Virus excretion in adults is associated with active disease. (Arrow = tubule with characteristic large cell containing intranuclear inclusion body.)

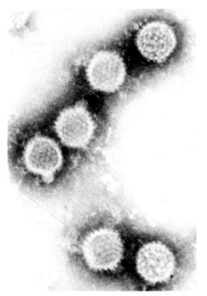

303

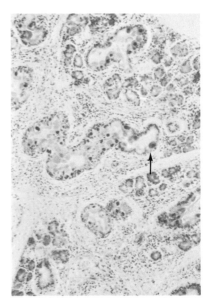

304

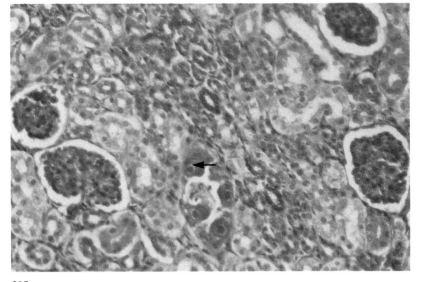

305

306 Radiograph of chest – cytomegalovirus infection in an immunodeficient patient. A high proportion of patients with renal or bone marrow transplants or with malignancies such as leukaemia or Hodgkin's disease develop active cytomegalovirus infection either because of primary infection or reactivation of latent infection. In many the infection remains subclinical; in others it may result in fever, infectious mononucleosis or pneumonitis. Cytomegalovirus infection of the lung is difficult to diagnose and may be associated with other opportunistic infections, such as candida and pneumocystis. Fever, dyspnoea and a non-productive cough are common among patients with serious pulmonary infection.

The radiological appearance of cytomegalovirus pneumonitis is not characteristic. In many patients there is an interstitial pattern of shadowing; in others there is a nodular pattern. The chest radiograph of this leukaemic child shows a large pneumatocele in the right lung caused by staphylococcal pneumonia, and diffuse interstitial shadowing caused by cytomegalovirus pneumonitis. The diagnosis was confirmed virologically.

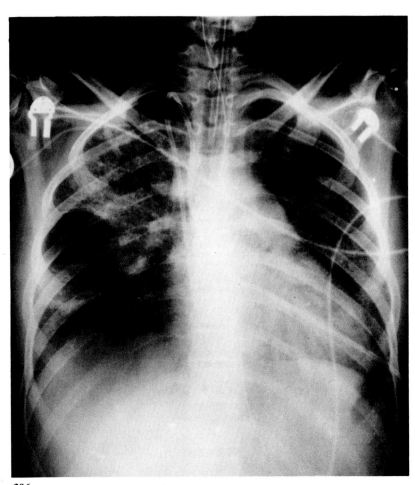

306

Infectious mononucleosis

Acute infectious mononucleosis is caused by Epstein–Barr virus (EBV), a herpesvirus with an affinity for lymphoid cells. It is a generalised disease which adopts many guises. The anginose variety is most commonly seen in young adults, but any organ may be affected, and clinical syndromes are not sharply demarcated. Characteristic changes are found in the patient's blood with a high proportion of abnormal mononuclear cells and many inappropriate antibodies. The diagnostic Paul–Bunnell–Davidsohn test detects a heterophile antibody, which agglutinates sheep red blood cells but is not absorbed by guinea-pig kidney. This test has to a large extent been supplanted by simplified variants. These heterophile antibody tests are usually positive during the acute stage of the illness, and antibody persists into convalescence: however, heterophile antibody tests may remain negative in approximately 10% of EBV infectious mononucleosis. Cytomegalovirus infection and toxoplasmosis may also present with a clinical syndrome of infectious mononucleosis.

The disease is endemic in most countries and has a striking predilection for young people between the ages of 15 and 20 years. The virus is transmitted by close contact with saliva from cases or carriers and there appear to be many subclinical infections, especially in young children. Studies of family or social contacts of patients with infectious mononucleosis have shown that spread occurs, but that infectivity is low. The incubation period is probably 33–49 days.

Virology and pathology

307 Electron micrograph of Epstein–Barr virus. EBV was originally detected in cells derived from Burkitt's lymphoma. It has the morphology of a herpesvirus with an electron-dense core of DNA. The virus may be recovered from throat swabs of patients with acute infectious mononucleosis and specific antibody may be detected in the IgM fraction of the patient's blood. EBV has also been implicated in nasopharyngeal carcinoma and has been associated with Hodgkin's disease, leukaemia and lymphoma.

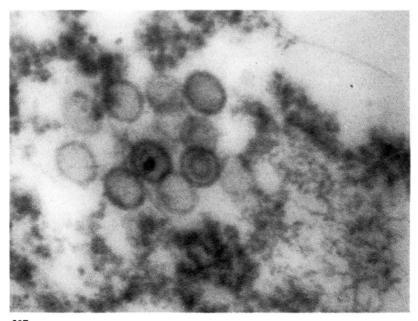

307

308 Blood film – abnormal mononuclear cells. The total white blood cell count is usually normal or slightly increased during the first week, but a few patients may have a neutropenia. A moderate leucocytosis develops towards the end of the first or the beginning of the second weeks, reaching a peak during the third. This leucocytosis is a result of an absolute increase in the circulating lymphocytes, many of which are abnormal. The virus is present in B lymphocytes.

The large number of atypical mononuclear cells found in the peripheral blood of patients with infectious mononucleosis is one of the characteristics of the disease. The cells vary greatly in size and shape. The nucleus may be round, bean-shaped, or lobulated; the cytoplasm is vacuolated and more basophilic than usual. Dividing cells are found in the peripheral blood, and mitotic activity is greatly enhanced, but cellular structure is not fundamentally deranged. The nuclear chromatin in most abnormal mononuclear cells is too coarse and the cytoplasm too abundant for confusion to arise with lymphoblasts.

Clinical features

309 Appearance of the face. Many patients with infectious mononucleosis have slight puffiness of the eyelids and a pinkish flush to their cheeks. When nasopharyngeal swelling (see **315**) is severe patients may have difficulty in breathing, which may progress to complete obstruction and respiratory failure.

310 Enanthem – petechiae. Various rashes have been found on the palate. A cluster of small haemorrhages at the junction of the hard and soft palate is almost invariably present in the anginose variety of infectious mononucleosis but is not pathognomonic, as similar lesions are found in other infections of the respiratory tract.

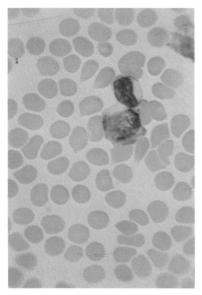

308

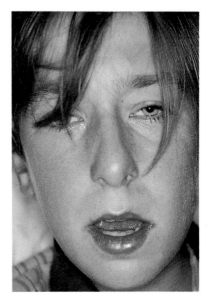

309

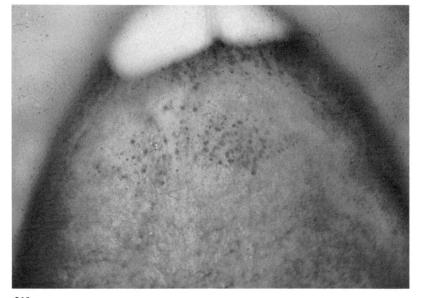

310

311 Anginose variety – inflamed throat without exudate. Shortly after onset of illness the patient may complain of a sore throat. The fauces are inflamed, but there is no exudate on the tonsils, and it is not possible from the appearance of the throat alone to make a diagnosis of infectious mononucleosis.

312 Anginose variety – follicular exudate. As the illness progresses patches of white exudate appear on the tonsils, which may be very swollen. The uvula is red and oedematous.

313 Anginose variety – typical exudate. The patches of exudate run together, forming thick plaques of opaque white membrane. The degree of inflammation varies considerably.

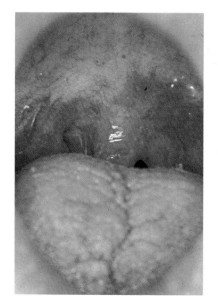

311

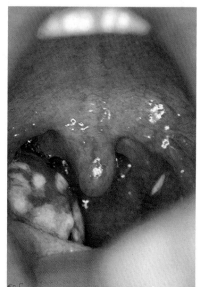

312

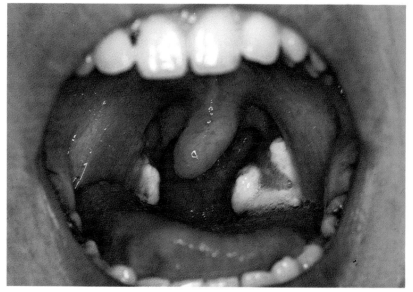

313

314 Anginose variety – late stage. The exudate persists for 7–14 days or even longer, and may completely cover both tonsils; however, the patient's general condition remains good. The membrane often retains its pristine whiteness as it matures, but the colour may alter. Note the enanthem on the palate.

315 Anginose variety – obstruction. In the most severe cases there may be so much congestion from inflammatory oedema that swallowing and breathing become difficult and life is endangered from respiratory obstruction.

It is difficult to recognise the normal anatomical landmarks. The tonsils are grossly swollen and covered with thick membrane, which obscures the uvula. The appearance of the throat might easily be mistaken for that caused by diphtheria, but the presence of splenomegaly and generalised enlargement of lymph nodes indicates the correct diagnosis. If doubt persists the matter can be settled by finding characteristic cells in the blood and a positive Paul–Bunnell test. If facilities for these tests are not available it would be advisable to give diphtheria antitoxin.

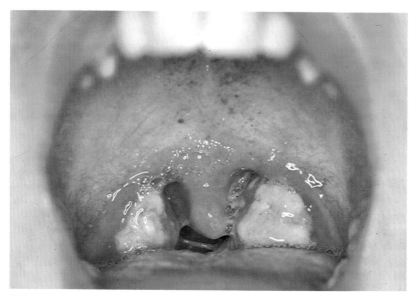

314

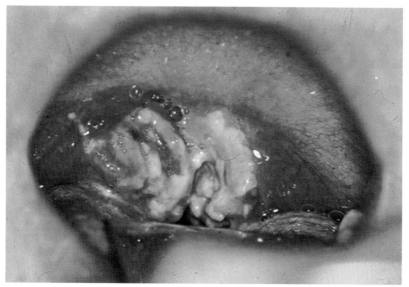

315

316 Rash on trunk. There is a high incidence of drug-related rashes among patients with infectious mononucleosis, but rashes also appear in those who have not been treated with drugs. The rash of infectious mononucleosis usually emerges during the second week, and with its pinkish maculopapular character may be mistaken for rubella. The duration of the prodromal period is a helpful guide.

317 Rash on upper limb. The distribution of the rash tends to be patchy and is heavier on the limbs. Contrast with the rash of rubella (**402–405**).

318 Ampicillin rash. The incidence of rashes is exceptionally high (at least 60%) in patients given ampicillin for the treatment of infectious mononucleosis. Drug-induced rashes are also common in patients receiving talampicillin and amoxycillin. The rashes are probably caused by sensitisation to polymers of these penicillins and are not indicative of allergy to other penicillins. This drug sensitivity is temporary and after a few months ampicillins can be used again safely.

The rash resembles that of measles but has a bluish tinge. The individual lesions may vary from one patient to another. Some lesions have a pale centre, others a dark centre.

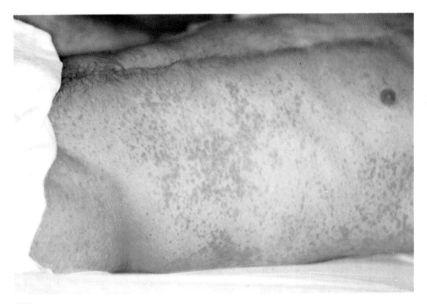

316

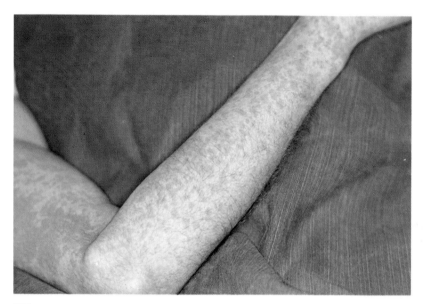

317

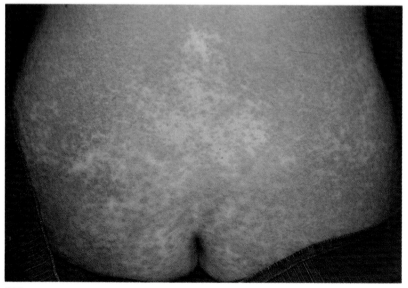

318

319 Ampicillin rash – close-up. Contrast with measles rash in **385**. Diagnosis is simple when exudate is present on the tonsils, but when exudate is absent there may be some confusion. The character of the individual components of the rash and the lack of respiratory catarrh exclude a diagnosis of measles.

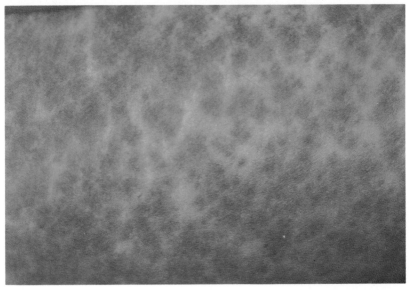

319

Viral hepatitis

Viral infections of the liver are particularly common throughout the world. An increasing number of viruses, currently designated A–E, have been identified with acute hepatitis. At least two types, hepatitis B and C, may become chronic and may lead to active chronic hepatitis, cirrhosis, and primary liver cancer. Less commonly, hepatitis is caused by other viruses, including yellow fever virus, cytomegalovirus, herpes simplex virus, and some strains of enteroviruses. A mild degree of hepatitis is also a very frequent finding in acute infectious mononucleosis.

Virus A hepatitis has a short incubation period of 28–42 days and predominantly affects children and young adults. The agent is an unenveloped single-stranded RNA virus, usually transmitted by the faecal–oral route. Several large outbreaks have been traced to water contaminated by sewage. Outbreaks caused by food-borne infection may result from direct contamination by a carrier, or indirectly from foodstuffs contaminated by infected water. In this respect shellfish are particularly dangerous. Many infections are subclinical. Young children tend to have anicteric attacks, presenting with mild gastrointestinal disturbance, whereas older children and adults become jaundiced. Hepatitis A has a relatively low mortality and chronic infection does not occur although abnormal liver function tests may persist for several months.

Hepatitis B has a long incubation period (6 weeks to 6 months) and is transmitted by body fluids, usually blood or sexual secretions. Babies may be infected *in utero* or during birth. In developed countries male homosexuals and intravenous drug abusers are the major groups at risk; in developing countries mother-to-baby spread maintains infection in the community, frequently resulting in chronic carriage of the virus rather than acute hepatitis. In parts of Africa and south-east Asia, where there is a high incidence of hepatitis B infection, primary liver cancer is common in adults of all ages. Those at particular risk appear to be chronic carriers of the virus, who were infected in early childhood. The cancer is commonly associated with hepatic cirrhosis. Primary liver cancer is thought to be the most common fatal neoplasm of humans. Morbidity and mortality rates of acute hepatitis B are greater than those of hepatitis A.

Hepatitis C is caused by a single-stranded RNA virus and is spread by the parenteral route. Half of those with acute hepatitis C progress to chronic hepatitis, at least one-fifth develop cirrhosis and a quarter terminate in liver failure.

Hepatitis D virus (delta agent) is an enveloped circular single-stranded RNA virus, which is parenterally transmitted. This virus is defective because it requires the presence of coincidental hepatitis B infection to produce hepatitis D. Alternatively, such dual infection may result in an especially severe form of hepatitis B.

Hepatitis E virus is an unenveloped single-stranded RNA virus, and is the second most important cause of faecal–oral spread of hepatitis after hepatitis virus A. It accounts for more than half of the cases of acute viral hepatitis in adults in many parts of the developing world. Large epidemics have occurred in developing countries and have affected mostly young and middle-aged adults – a particularly high mortality rate of 20–39% has been seen in pregnant women.

Virology and pathology

320 Electron micrograph of a negatively stained preparation of virus B hepatitis serum. Serum from patients with hepatitis B has been found to contain three distinct particles – Dane particles, spheres and tubules. All three are agglutinated by antiserum to hepatitis B surface antigen (HBsAg). The larger, double-shelled, Dane particle is believed to be the virus and structures similar to the inner core have been detected in the liver of patients with acute hepatitis. The amorphous spheres and tubules appear to be incomplete particles of viral coat. During the early stage of hepatitis the particles are evenly dispersed, but as the illness progresses they clump together with antibody to form large immune complexes. In chronic carriers the particles remain discrete.

HBsAg has been found in most body fluids but only serum, saliva, and semen are infectious. HBsAg appears in the circulation after an incubation period of 1–3 months and can be detected for a few weeks in self-limiting infections; it may persist indefinitely in carriers of the virus. The production of antibody to HBsAg (anti-HBs) is very variable in relation to clearance of HBsAg. Anti-HBs formed as a result of virus B infection or following immunisation confers immunity.

HBsAg varies in antigenic structure and has at least eight sub-types. These variations have proved useful in epidemiological studies. Hepatitis B core antigen (HBcAg) is present in the nucleus of infected hepatocytes and is present in the circulation only as an internal component of the Dane particle. Anti-HBc can usually be detected 3–5 weeks after HBsAg appears in serum, and persists throughout the clinical illness and for several years afterwards. Anti-HBc is not formed after immunisation. HBeAg in serum is associated with a high concentration of Dane particles and is a marker of infectivity. HBsAg is comparatively rare among the general population of western Europe and North America, and is more commonly found in Japan and many tropical countries. (A = Dane particle, B = tubule, C = sphere.)

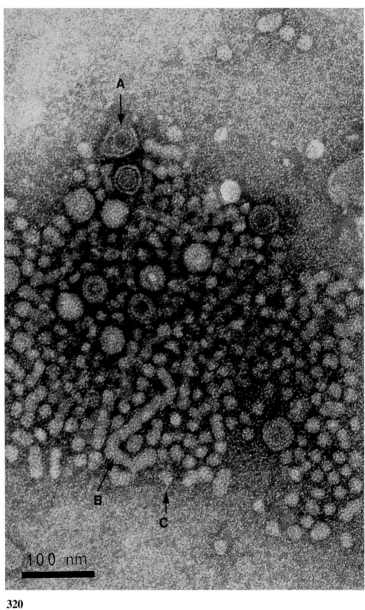

320

321 Histology of acute hepatitis (haematoxylin and eosin stain). There are no differences in the appearance of the liver in the two main types of viral hepatitis. The entire liver is affected, and the degree of impairment corresponds roughly to the severity of the histological changes.

During the acute stage parenchymal cells in any part of the liver may undergo necrosis. The affected cells are shrunken and rounded, with an intensely eosinophilic cytoplasm. The nucleus degenerates and disappears, leaving a globular eosinophilic structure. In the regions most distant from the portal tracts the liver cells become swollen, the nuclei disintegrate, and the affected cells disappear.

The Küpffer cells enlarge and increase in number. There is heavy infiltration with lymphocytes, plasma cells and histiocytes round the portal tracts. In uncomplicated cases the Küpffer cell reaction begins to subside after a month, and the inflammatory reaction in the portal tracts has disappeared by the end of 2 months. The normal structure of the liver is fully restored.

In the section shown here the architecture of the liver is intact. A dying liver cell is easily recognised in the centre of the picture by its eosinophilic appearance and pyknotic nucleus. The Küpffer cells are prominent, but at this early stage there is little infiltration by inflammatory cells. (A = degenerate hepatocyte with pyknotic nucleus, B = Küpffer cells.)

322 Chronic persistent hepatitis. Section of liver (haematoxylin and eosin stain). Occasionally, mild symptoms may persist for more than a year after an acute attack of hepatitis, and the liver remains enlarged with a normal or firm consistency. Minor abnormalities are usually found on liver function tests.

On biopsy the liver characteristically has a normal reticulin framework, but there is conspicuous round cell infiltration of the portal tracts and patchy necrosis of the liver cells. Although the histological appearance may remain unaltered for years, the outcome is generally favourable, with minimal scarring in the portal zones. Very rarely, the process terminates in cirrhosis.

In the section shown here a dense pattern of round cells and fibrous cells is seen in the portal tract. Some of the parenchymal cells show evidence of incipient necrosis with darkly stained cytoplasm and pyknotic nuclei. (A = portal tract, B = parenchyma.)

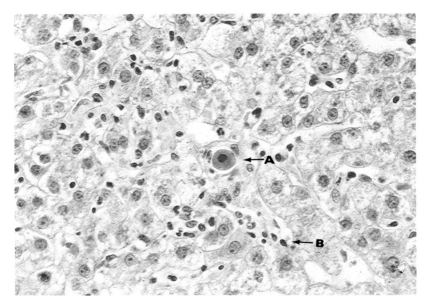

321

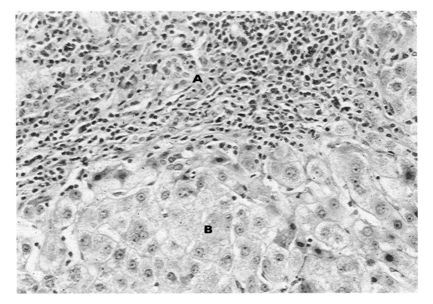

322

323 Hepatic necrosis. Histology of liver (haematoxylin and eosin stain). In a few patients with severe hepatitis, recovery may be accompanied by extensive scarring. During the acute stage of the illness widespread destruction of parenchymal cells leads to collapse of the reticulin framework and approximation of adjacent portal tracts. As recovery takes place the destroyed liver cells are replaced by fibrous tissue, which separates nodules of regenerated liver cells. With time, the fibrous tissue contracts and becomes less cellular. The final stage is a coarsely scarred nodular liver.

The section shows an early stage of the process with a band of fibrous tissue and lymphocytes separating nodules of parenchymal cells. (A = fibrous tissue and lymphocytes, B = parenchymal cells.)

Clinical features

324 Appearance of urine in hepatitis. In acute viral hepatitis bilirubin appears in the urine before the patient becomes jaundiced. Urobilin is found in the urine during the early stages but disappears at the height of the illness and returns as liver function improves.

Urine containing bile is greenish or brownish-yellow in colour. The surface tension is altered and froth, which forms on top after shaking, is usually permanent. Conjugated billirubin is excreted in the urine but unconjugated bilirubin is not. Urine containing an excess of urobilin develops a warm orange colour on standing.

The colour of the faeces in virus hepatitis varies with the degree of intrahepatic obstruction.

325 Jaundiced sclera. Elastic tissue has a special affinity for bilirubin, so structures with a high content of elastic tissue, such as skin, ocular sclera and blood vessels, readily become jaundiced and retain the pigment even after the serum bilirubin has returned to normal.

Compare the jaundiced eye of viral hepatitis with the suffused eye of leptospiral jaundice in **176**.

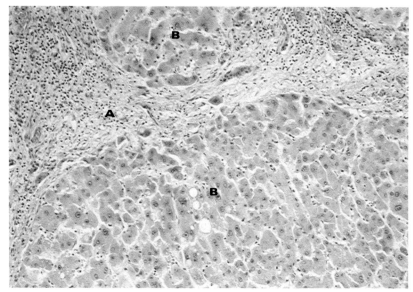

323

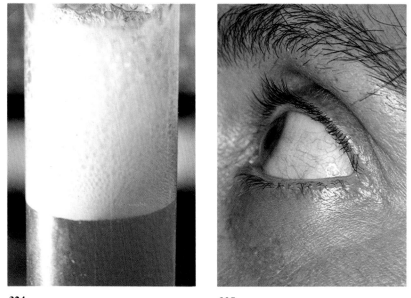

324

325

326 Jaundiced skin. The water-soluble conjugated bilirubin, found in patients with hepatocellular and cholestatic jaundice, produces a more intense colour in the skin than the unconjugated pigment of haemolytic jaundice. The skin of patients with long-standing obstructive jaundice may have a greenish tinge, possibly as a result of biliverdin and other pigments.

In this illustration the colour of normal skin is contrasted with the yellow skin of a patient with acute hepatitis.

327 Rash in viral hepatitis. Rashes are found in 5% of patients with viral hepatitis. They are seen more commonly in HBsAg-positive hepatitis, particularly in the preicteric phase, when they may be associated with arthralgia. The rash may be erythematous, maculopapular, or urticarial. Purpuric rashes are common in patients with liver failure.

The illustration shows an erythematous rash on the leg of a patient with virus B hepatitis.

328 Virus B hepatitis. Long-incubation (virus B) hepatitis is generally transmitted by blood or blood products. As little as 0.004 ml of serum has been known to cause infection. Patients and staff in renal dialysis units are particularly vulnerable to this disease, and there is also a high incidence in drug addicts and homosexuals.

The patient shown here was one of a group of young men infected from a tattooing needle. The intensity of the jaundice is shown by the contrast with the normal colour of the physician's hand.

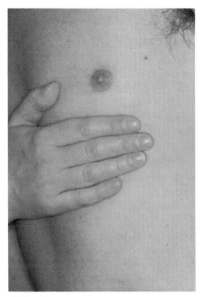

326

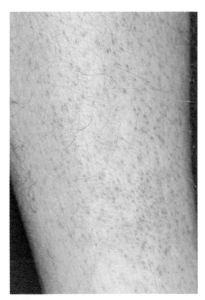

327

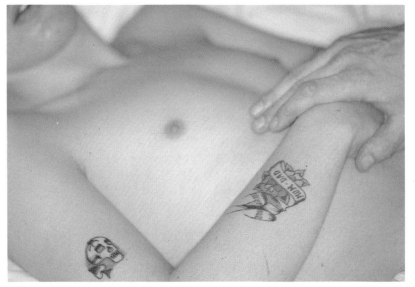

328

Human immune deficiency virus (HIV) infection

The acquired immune deficiency syndrome (AIDS) was first described in 1981 and the causative virus, human immune deficiency virus (HIV 1) identified 2 years later. Subsequently another virus was recognised in West African patients with AIDS-like syndrome; this virus, although designated HIV 2, more closely resembles a simian retrovirus. The origin of these viruses is obscure, although they may have evolved from related simian viruses.

After entering the body HIV attaches itself to CD4 antigen on the surface membrane of some cells, particularly helper (T4) lymphocytes but also other cells, notably mononuclear and microglial. Within the cell viral RNA is transformed by the viral enzyme, reverse transcriptase, into DNA and incorporated into the host cell chromosomes, where it remains latent until activated to produce fresh virus particles. Viruses with the ability to convert RNA to DNA in this manner are designated retroviruses.

As HIV infection progresses cell-mediated immunity wanes, predisposing the patient to infection with predominantly intracellular pathogens and to the development of certain neoplasms, particularly Kaposi's sarcoma and non-Hodgkin's lymphoma. Humoral immunity is also affected because polyclonal stimulation of B lymphocytes results in the production of antibodies that are mostly inappropriate to host defences.

Defective immunity has many consequences. In most infections an intact immune system is necessary for the development of the classical clinical features of disease. If immunity is deficient clinical presentation may be atypical and antibody tests used for diagnosis may be misleading. Moreover, when immunity is deficient multiple infections are not uncommon.

329 Electron micrograph of HIV.

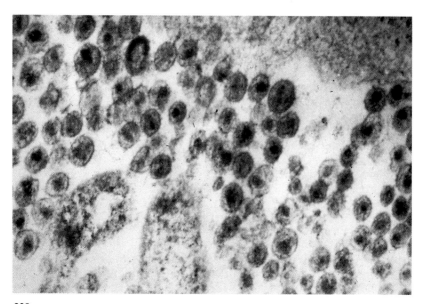

329

330 Intravenous drug track marks. HIV may be transmitted by sexual contact, by blood and blood products, and from infected mother to fetus or infant. Homosexual transmission is common in North America, western Europe and Australia giving a male:female ratio of 15:1; heterosexual transmission is common in sub-Saharan Africa, with a male:female ratio of about 1:1. Many haemophiliacs and recipients of blood transfusions were infected before donor screening and heat treatment of clotting factors were introduced in 1985. Transmission by sharing needles and equipment contaminated by blood gave rise to rapid spread in intravenous drug abusers (IVDA). Infection may also be spread by reused, inadequately sterilised surgical equipment and needles or other skin-penetrating instruments. Prevalence of HIV infection in children is high in areas where much spread is by intravenous drug abuse.

Marks on the skin caused by injection of caustic or contaminated drugs are a sure sign of current intravenous drug abuse and its attendant infection risks, including HIV, hepatitis B and C, septicaemia, and endocarditis. Because the interval from infection with HIV to AIDS is about 10 years, most patients presenting with AIDS acquired by intravenous drug abuse will have abandoned the practice and no longer have such stigmata.

331 The illness of infection (seroconversion illness) – skin rash. This develops about 6 weeks after invasion by HIV and occurs at the time of seroconversion. It presents as an infectious mononucleosis-like illness with fever, sore throat, lymph node enlargement, muscle pains, and a variety of rashes. In some instances there may be a mild self-limiting encephalitis.

Most people do not have an illness at the time of seroconversion and some may remain well for several years. Others may develop acute aseptic meningitis at the time of seroconversion, or encephalitis with diffuse or focal signs may appear during the period of 3 months following conversion. Thereafter, many patients may remain symptom-free for about 10 years, although there may be persistent lymph node enlargement. At the end of this latent period some develop the characteristic features of AIDS with opportunistic infections or neoplasms; others may present with AIDS-related complex (ARC), a term applied to a nonspecific illness lacking diagnostic features of the fully developed syndrome.

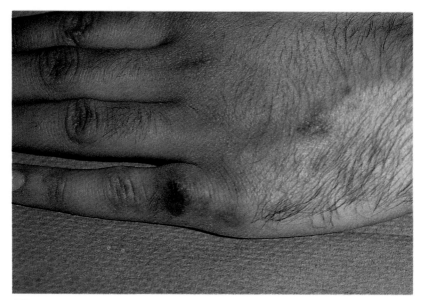

330

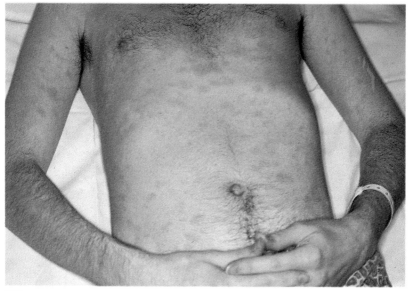

331

332 Seborrhoeic dermatitis. This form of dermatitis is a very common condition in patients with AIDS and is associated with low-grade, non-candidal fungal infection.

333 Oral hairy leukoplakia. This condition is caused by combined infection with HIV and Epstein–Barr virus. It is found in the late stage of persistent HIV infection and in most cases will be followed by AIDS within 2 years. Oral hairy leukoplakia is only rarely found in immunodeficiency due to other causes.

The name is derived from the microscopic appearance of the leukoplakia. HIV-related leukoplakia consists of raised white areas of thickening usually present on both sides of the tongue. In this situation the continuity of the leukoplakia is interrupted by vertical grooves, giving a corrugated appearance. Leukoplakia may also be found on the dorsum or ventral surfaces of the tongue, the buccal mucosa, the floor of the mouth, or the palate. In these sites the lesions are flat and non-corrugated. Usually the condition is symptom-free and treatment is unnecessary.

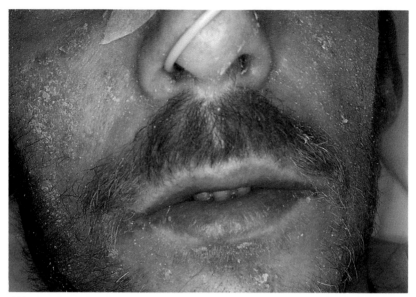

332

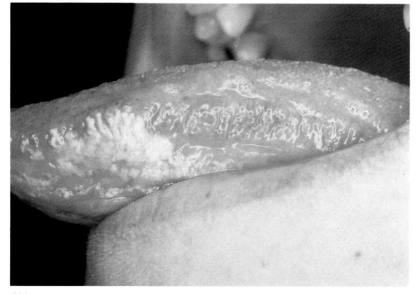

333

277

334 Herpes simplex. Latent herpes simplex virus may reactivate when cell-mediated immunity is depressed by disease or treatment (see **300**). In HIV infection with persistent immunodeficiency, repeated reactivation of the virus may take place. The resulting eruptions may have the classic appearance of herpes simplex with clusters of vesicles but in HIV-related immunodeficiency the classic presentation is frequently modified as vesicles merge into each other before rupturing and creating areas of superficial ulceration.

In male homosexuals repeated reactivation of genital herpes may be a major problem, especially if the virus damages the ganglia of sacral nerves. In this situation bladder and bowel function may be impaired.

335 Herpes zoster. As immunity following an attack of varicella wanes, reactivation of virus latent in nerve ganglia results in an attack of herpes zoster (see **243** and **244**). This may happen early in the course of HIV infection, when immunodeficiency is mild, and several years may elapse before an AIDS-defining illness develops. At this stage the immune response is usually sufficient to control the herpes zoster and further episodes are uncommon. Because the incidence of herpes zoster is higher in patients with HIV infection than in age-matched members of the general population, an attack of herpes zoster in a young adult with no predisposing factors is unusual and should always arouse suspicion of an underlying HIV infection. Should an attack of herpes zoster affect a patient with established AIDS several dermatomes may be involved. In this event viral activity may continue unchecked and the lesions fail to heal.

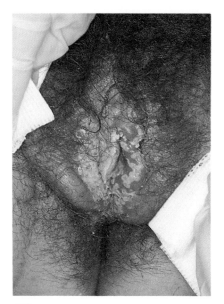

334

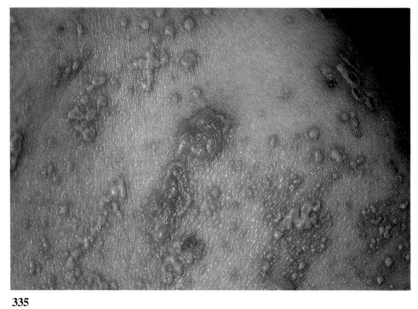

335

279

336 Oral thrush. This is an early sign of immunosuppression. In patients with normal immunity candida produces discrete patches of thrush (see **130**); in patients with HIV infection oral thrush tends to be more extensive with multiple small patches, or larger patches exceeding 1 cm in diameter .

337 Candida oesophagitis – barium swallow. Painful dysphagia in the presence of oral thrush strongly suggests candida oesophagitis, which is an AIDS-defining condition.

Plaques of thrush accompanied by diffuse ulceration of the oesophageal mucosa produce a characteristic cobblestone appearance on radiographic examination after a barium swallow. This differs from the appearance produced by cytomegalovirus oesophagitis, which is commonly associated with large shallow ulcers. In contrast, herpes simplex oesophagitis gives rise to multiple deep ulcers.

338 Tinea. Fungal infections of the skin may proceed unchecked and be more florid or less typical than usual. Tinea (ringworm) may be widespread in multiple small patches or confined to a single large area.

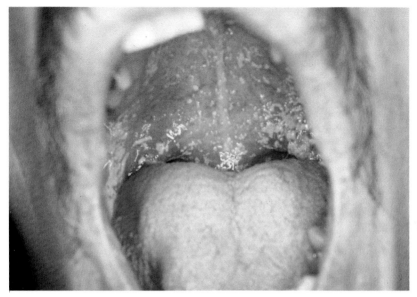

336

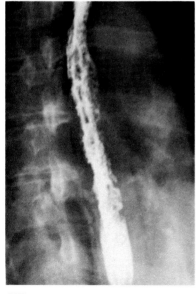

337

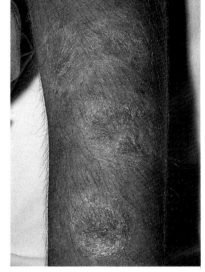

338

339 Pneumocystis pneumonia – radiograph of chest. *Pneumocystis carinii* pneumonia (PCP) is a common AIDS-defining illness, especially in intravenous drug abusers. The onset is usually insidious, with excessive tiredness. After a few weeks the patient becomes progressively dyspnoeic and may develop a persistent non-productive cough. In the early stage the chest radiograph may be normal; at a later stage patchy shadowing develops, which may spare the lung apices and bases. Even when the appearance of the chest radiograph is normal, blood gas analysis commonly reveals notable hypoxia. It is not possible to make a diagnosis from the radiographic appearance, and microscopy, using immuno-fluorescent techniques on sputum or bronchiolar lavage, is usually necessary to confirm the aetiology of the pneumonia.

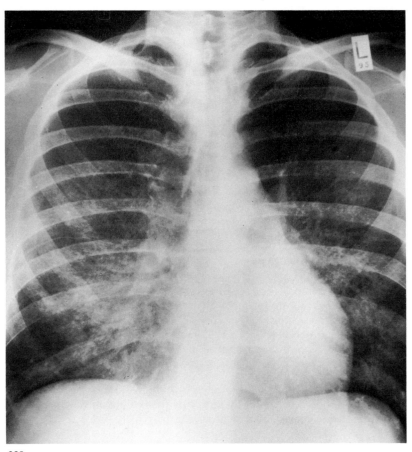

339

283

340 Pneumocystis pneumonia – histology of lung (haematoxylin and eosin stain). *Pneumocystis carinii* was at one time classified as a protozoon but is now believed to be a fungus. It is frequently found in animals and not uncommonly in humans. Human infection is usually latent but the organism may give rise to interstitial plasma cell pneumonia, particularly in premature babies, or in older children or adults with chronic debilitating diseases or disorders of immunity. Pneumocystis infection is particularly common in children with thymic aplasia. Fatal pneumonia has occasionally occurred as a primary illness. The mode of transmission is uncertain, but small outbreaks among neonates have suggested that infection may be airborne. Pneumocystis pneumonia is a very common presentation of AIDS and may occur alone or in conjunction with other opportunistic infections such as cytomegalovirus, mycobacteria, or cryptococcus.

At necropsy the lungs are distended, and the cut surfaces grey and airless. The interlobular septa are thickened and infiltrated with histiocytes, lymphocytes, and plasma cells. The alveoli are distended with a foamy, semi-liquid substance – when suitably stained this is found to be teeming with organisms. Plasma cells may be diminished in number or absent in patients with agammaglobulinaemia or hypogammaglobulinaemia. (A = alveolus distended with foamy material, B = histiocyte, C = plasma cell, D = lymphocyte.)

341 *Pneumocystis carinii* pneumonia (Grocott's silver-impregnation stain). The parasite is found in the lungs as a small cyst, containing two to eight unnucleated bodies. These are very small, measuring 2–4 μm in length, and are oval or crescent shaped. The organism divides by binary fission. It may be stained by many dyes but not with haematoxylin and eosin.

342 *Pneumocystis carinii* demonstrated by immunofluorescence. The parasite is most readily detected for diagnostic purposes using immunofluorescent techniques on sputum or specimens obtained by bronchiolar lavage.

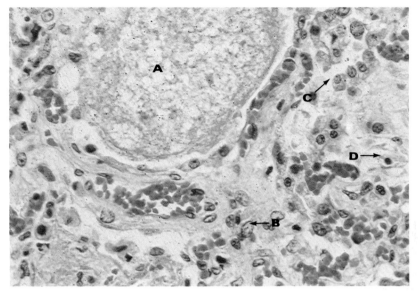

340

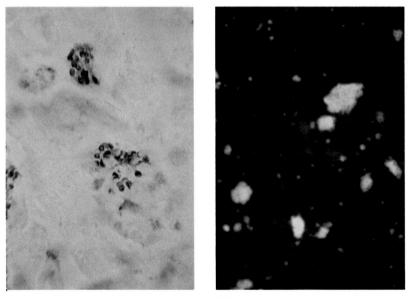

341

342

343 AIDS and cytomegalovirus infection. Section of kidney showing inclusion bodies. Cytomegalovirus (CMV) infection is very common in those who have acquired HIV sexually. In HIV-positive patients with an active CMV infection the virus may be found in almost any tissue. In late-stage HIV infection, CMV may be isolated from the throat or urine of nearly all those infected with CMV. However, it should be appreciated that the isolation of CMV does not necessarily indicate that it is responsible for any symptoms the patient might have. To confirm that such isolates are relevant to the illness it is necessary to detect diagnostic changes on fundoscopy or to find characteristic histological appearances on biopsy of relevant tissues (see **303–5**).

344 Cytomegalovirus retinitis. CMV retinitis is the most common cause of loss of vision in AIDS patients and is the AIDS-defining illness in 1–2% of HIV-positive patients.

CMV retinitis usually develops at a late stage of AIDS, when CD4 counts are below 50 cells/mm^3. The typical appearances have been memorably described as 'bushfire, ketchup, and cottage cheese': the perivascular waxy exudates resemble cottage cheese; haemorrhages in the surrounding area ketchup; the haemorrhages round the edges but less marked in the centre of the lesions have been likened to bushfire. The initial lesions are usually unilateral but spread to the other eye in about 60% of cases. Although some of the retinal lesions may not deteriorate, CMV retinitis may sometimes progress so rapidly that immediate treatment is essential to prevent blindness.

345 Cytomegalovirus encephalitis – magnetic resonance scan. CMV may cause other neurological abnormalities, including meningoencephalitis, myelopathies, polyradiculitis, and neuropathy. CMV encephalitis is difficult to diagnose without biopsy and, even if confirmed, may be associated with other opportunistic infections or with lymphoma.

Magnetic resonance scans may be normal or show low-density focal lesions in the white matter, in the subependymal periventricular areas, or in the cortex. Administration of contrast, which highlights areas of increased blood supply, gives variable results depending on the vascularity of the affected area.

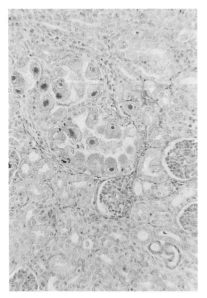

343

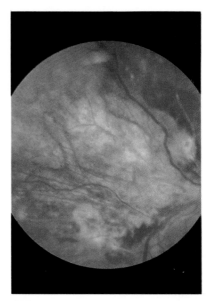

344

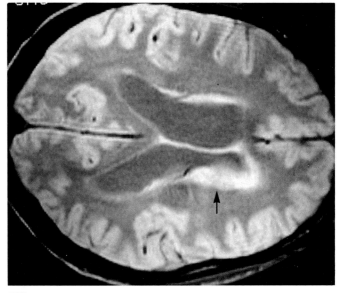

345

346 Cerebral toxoplasmosis – magnetic resonance scan. Toxoplasma encephalitis, 'brain abscess', is the most common intracerebral space-occupying lesion in AIDS. The prevalence of toxoplasmosis varies in different parts of the world and this is reflected in the varying incidence of toxoplasmosis infections in patients with AIDS. In France up to 25% of AIDS patients will develop active toxoplasmosis, whereas only 4–5% in the USA will do so.

AIDS patients with cerebral toxoplasmosis usually present with a hemiplegia, fits, visual disturbance or impaired mental function, suggesting the possibility of multiple space-occupying lesions. Computed tomography (CT) scans or magnetic resonance (MR) scans are usually abnormal, with multiple circular lesions of variable size. Ring enhancement associated with surrounding hyperaemia and oedema is found in 90% of lesions and is prominent after the administration of contrast media. Serological tests may not be helpful in establishing the diagnosis because specific IgM antibody may not be present if the organism has been acutely reactivated. IgG antibody will confirm that the patient has been infected with toxoplasma *at some time* but does not prove that infection is active. Failure of the lesions to shrink on effective treatment with appropriate drugs makes a diagnosis of uncomplicated cerebral toxoplasmosis unlikely and other possibilities, such as CMV or cryptococcal infection, or lymphoma, should be considered.

347 Toxoplasma retinitis. Areas of necrosis may be found in the retina but haemorrhages are unusual. At an early stage clusters of yellowish cotton-wool spots appear on the retina. These may coalesce to form larger lesions, which have a punched-out appearance and evoke little or no vitreous reaction. The retinitis may result in visual field defects. With healing the lesions become atrophic, and black pigmentation may be a prominent feature.

348 Cotton-wool spots. These spots are not uncommon in AIDS patients and, if caused by HIV, may disappear from time to time. They are usually asymptomatic. Because CMV or toxoplasma retinitis may also begin with insignificant lesions on the retina they may be overlooked, so it is essential that cotton-wool spots are reviewed regularly by an expert ophthalmologist.

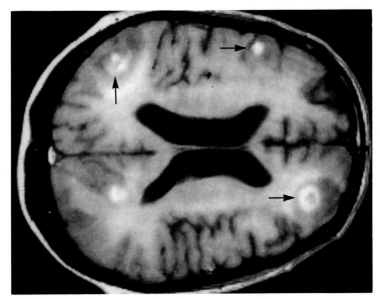

346

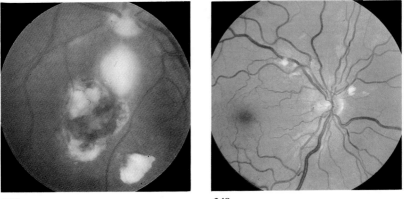

347

348

349 HIV encephalopathy – magnetic resonance scan. When HIV encephalopathy develops early it manifests clinically with memory loss, impaired concentration, and mental slowing. CT scans show generalised atrophy of the brain in 70–90% of patients, and MR scans reveal that the abnormalities are mostly in the subcortical white matter. When encephalopathy appears at a later stage it is more dramatic with marked cognitive abnormalities, memory loss, behaviour change, and psychomotor impairment. Scans then reveal extreme cerebral atrophy with loss of brain volume, widened sulci, ventricular dilatation, and abnormalities in the white matter.

350 Cryptosporidiosis – direct smear of stool (Ziehl-Neelsen stain). Cryptosporidiosis is a protozoal infection of the bowel derived from domestic or food animals, or from infected individuals, especially children. Infection may be spread by contaminated food or water. In otherwise healthy individuals cryptosporidiosis is a benign infection causing a self-limiting attack of gastroenteritis; in AIDS patients it may cause intractable diarrhoea or invade the biliary tract, giving rise to cholangitis or cholecystitis. Striking histological changes may be apparent in the gut of AIDS patients, with severe inflammation and even gangrene. The diagnosis is established by detecting oocysts in a direct smear of stool stained by modified Ziehl-Neelsen, auramine or Giemsa. It may be necessary to concentrate the stool specimen.

351 Slim disease. This name has been given by the resident population in parts of rural Africa to the severe wasting disease found in HIV-positive individuals. Marked weight loss is accompanied by profound fatigue, feverishness, sweating and diarrhoea. As a rule there is no evidence of neoplasia or opportunistic infections. Patients with slim disease waste away and die from a combination of malnutrition and secondary infections. The cause of this syndrome is not fully understood. It may be caused by a general direct action of HIV leading to failure of multiple organs, or it may be the consequence of an unrecognised opportunistic infection peculiar to Africa.

An unexplained constitutional disturbance for more than a month with a temperature exceeding 38°C, associated with diarrhoea and an otherwise unexplained loss of more than 10% of body weight, is an AIDS-defining syndrome in any HIV-positive patient.

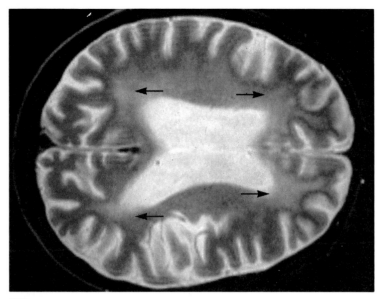

349

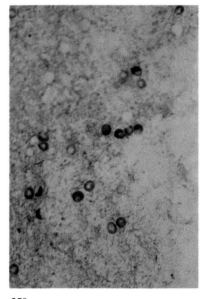

350

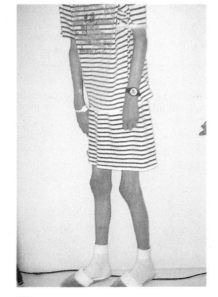

351

352 Progressive multifocal leukoencephalopathy – magnetic resonance scan. Progressive multifocal leukoencephalopathy (PML) is a progressive demyelinating central nervous system disease caused by JC papovavirus. PML is found in 2–7% of AIDS patients. The disease evolves rapidly and results in death within 2–4 months.

Symptoms are varied, depending on the sites of demyelination, and include limb weakness, personality changes, mental impairment, ataxia, dysarthria, and cortical blindness. Quadriplegia and coma commonly precede death.

MR scanning shows diffuse areas of low density in the white matter, which do not enhance after contrast is given. (Ring enhancement around multiple lesions suggests toxoplasmosis.) Definitive diagnosis requires brain biopsy. Serological tests are unhelpful because antibodies to JC virus can be detected in the serum of most normal adults.

353 Cerebral lymphoma – magnetic resonance scan. Non-Hodgkin's lymphoma is, after Kaposi's sarcoma, the second most common HIV-related malignancy and is found in 2–5% of AIDS patients. This lymphoma is derived from B lymphocytes and is highly aggressive. Although non-Hodgkin's lymphoma can affect many sites it has a tendency to present as a space-occupying cerebral lesion. Symptoms include limb weakness, cranial nerve palsies, headache, and epileptic fits.

On MR scanning non-Hodgkin's lymphoma, in contrast to toxoplasmosis, usually appears as a single lesion, although there may be closely related groups of lesions. The centres of the lesions may be dense or necrotic. Diagnosis is usually made on brain biopsy. Lumbar puncture is generally contraindicated when a space-occupying lesion is found on scanning. Occasionally, cerebral lymphoma may present with diffuse meningeal involvement. In this event, if a lumbar puncture is performed, the cerebrospinal fluid should be examined for mycobacteria and fungi, and any lymphocytes examined for markers of malignancy.

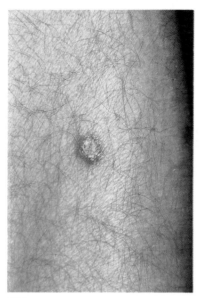

354

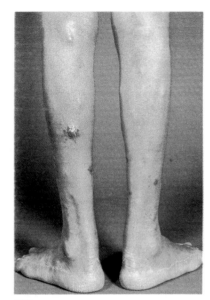

355

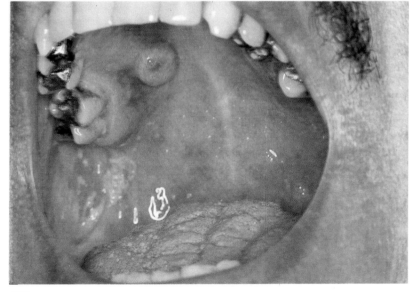

356

357 *Cryptococcus neoformans* (**nigrosin stain**). *Cryptococcus neoformans* is a true yeast that reproduces by budding and does not form mycelia. The cells are spherical in shape and measure 5–20 µm in diameter. The organism is Gram positive and has a thick gelatinous capsule, which is clearly visible in Indian ink or nigrosin preparations. Cryptococci grow slowly on selective media, such as Sabouraud's glucose agar or tellurite malt agar. Pathogenicity can be established by inoculating mice.

C. neoformans causes sporadic infections in humans and animals. The source of infection in humans is uncertain, but the yeast is commonly present in mammals and birds, and withstands drying in soil and dust. Pigeon droppings are the most abundant known source of virulent strains. The mode of transmission is equally uncertain but it is likely that the organism gains access through the respiratory or alimentary tracts.

358 **Cryptococcal meningitis and AIDS.** The cryptococcus rarely causes trouble in healthy individuals, in whom it may be found on the skin or in the bowel contents. Pulmonary infection is often a benign incidental finding. Patients with reticuloses and AIDS are especially vulnerable to cryptococcal meningitis. The incidence of cryptococcal infection in AIDS patients depends on the presence of the organism in the environment. In the USA cryptococcal infection is found in 10% of AIDS patients. In most of those infected the cryptococcus is present in the bloodstream and 80% develop signs of meningitis.

Cryptococcal disease of the brain and meninges usually follows a subacute or chronic course with a very high mortality. The presenting features are non-specific with malaise, fever, sweating and vague headache; as the illness progresses the headache becomes more severe and signs of meningitis appear. Focal neurological phenomena, such as epileptic fits and limb weakness, are rare. The diagnosis is established by finding the organism in the cerebrospinal fluid or by demonstrating the presence of cryptococcal antigen.

Cryptococci may invade tissues and multiply by budding without initially provoking an inflammatory reaction, but eventually their presence in larger numbers leads to infiltration with round cells and macrophages. Granulomatous lesions form and are conspicuous around the base of the brain. In this section of the cerebral cortex arrows point to capsulated spheroidal cryptococci.

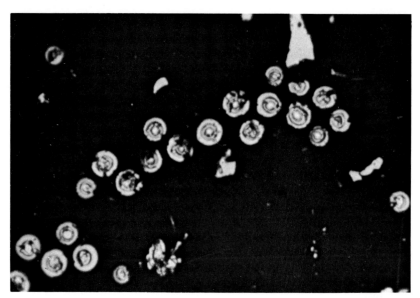

357

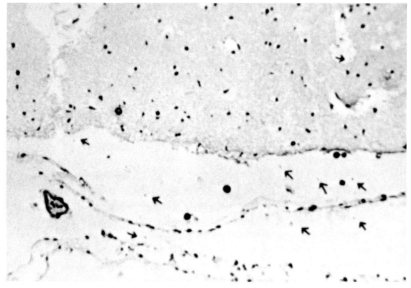

358

Myxovirus infection

Myxoviruses are responsible for many respiratory diseases in humans, other mammals, and birds. They are so named because they possess a special affinity for mucin. The viruses contain a core of RNA, with protein capsomeres arranged along its coils. The outer membrane has a lipid component, so the viruses are sensitive to ether. Most myxoviruses possess haemagglutinins, and some also possess haemolysins. The viruses are easily deformed and therefore difficult to measure, but commonly range in size from 80 to 150 nm. They may be spherical or filamentous in shape. Myxoviruses can be divided into two subgroups, but only those members affecting humans will be considered.

(a) Orthomyxoviruses – influenza viruses A, B, and C. These are small and have filamentous forms. The internal structure of RNA is slender. They lack haemolysins.

(b) Paramyxoviruses – measles virus, mumps virus, parainfluenza viruses 1, 2, 3, and 4. These are large and vary in size. The RNA structure is thicker. Filamentous forms are not found. They possess haemolysins as well as haemagglutinins.

Influenza

Influenza is a highly infectious disease caused by *Myxovirus influenzae*. There are three distinct serotypes (A, B, and C), each containing antigenic strains. Virus strains are designated according to their type, geographic origin, strain number, and year first isolated, e.g. A/Hong Kong/1/68. Although the illness caused by influenza A and B cannot be distinguished clinically, the epidemiological pattern is different. Virus A causes both pandemics and localised outbreaks, affecting all age groups, and is associated with high mortality in the elderly and those with pre-existing cardiac or pulmonary disease. Virus B is found in sporadic cases and in limited epidemics, especially institutional outbreaks in young people. It tends to cause milder disease and has been linked with Reye's syndrome. Virus C is probably not a human pathogen. Infection is derived from the nasal and pharyngeal secretions of human cases and is spread by the airborne route to the respiratory passages.

A short incubation period of 1–4 days is followed by abrupt onset of fever with headache and myalgia. The virus damages the respiratory mucosa, causing nasal obstruction, sore throat, and a dry hacking cough. Sweating is a prominent feature. In uncomplicated influenza there are few physical signs. The duration of the illness is very variable, but the temperature usually returns to normal on the third or fourth day. Recovery tends to be slow and postinfluenzal depression common. In severe attacks bronchiolitis and pneumonia may be caused directly by the virus or may result from secondary bacterial invasion of the lungs. Although mortality is low, the attack rate is high and pandemics caused by a new antigenic strain may result in millions of deaths.

Virology

359   Electron micrograph of influenza virus. Particles from infected allantoic fluid are spherical in shape and measure 80–120 nm in diameter. Recently isolated virus A may be filamentous and measure several microns in length but have the same diameter. The virions consists of a hollow, helically arranged RNA thread, 8000 nm in length and 9 nm in diameter, coiled in a central mass. This viral nucleoprotein is formed within the nucleus of the host cell. The lipid envelope has rod-like projections containing two antigens, H (haemagglutination) and N (neuraminidase). Antigenic drift results from minor changes within the H antigen, and antigenic shift is due to genetic recombination during replication, which permits the emergence of an antigenically different virus with new proteins constituting either or both of H and N antigens. Epidemics are associated with antigenic drift; pandemics may follow antigenic shift.

Influenza viruses can be grown on embryonated hen eggs and cultures of mammalian cells. The virus causes agglutination of human and fowl red blood cells. Each type of influenza virus is characterised by its specific nucleoprotein (soluble) antigen. Antigens in the envelope (V antigens H and N) give subtype or strain-specific reactions.

Pathology

360   Section of trachea (haematoxylin and eosin stain). The trachea and bronchi bear the brunt of the initial damage to the respiratory tract by influenza virus. The submucosa is swollen and infiltrated by mononuclear cells, while the ciliated columnar layer has been shed from the basement membrane. This injury to the lining of the trachea and bronchi paves the way for secondary invasion by bacteria from the upper respiratory passages.

(A = desquamating epithelium, B = basement membrane, C = submucosa with mononuclear cells, D = cartilage ring.)

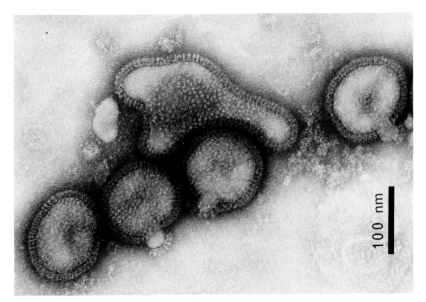

359

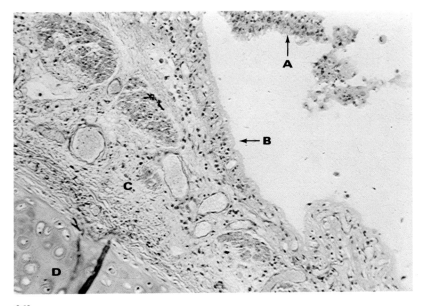

360

When death occurs during the early stages of influenza, before secondary bacterial invasion, the lungs are brightly mottled with subpleural haemorrhages, and blood-stained fluid runs freely from any cut surface. On section the lungs are haemorrhagic and solid, a finding that readily explains the extreme respiratory distress and cyanosis preceding death. Pneumonia developing at a later stage is caused by secondary bacterial infection, frequently staphylococcal.

361   Section of lung in influenza (haematoxylin and eosin stain). The alveolar walls are thickened and infiltrated by mononuclear cells. The air sacs are free from exudate. there is congestion around the small bronchus in the centre of the section, and the lumen is plugged with mononuclear cells. (A = air sac, B = thickened alveolar wall, C = bronchus with plug.)

362   Section of lung in influenza (haematoxylin and eosin stain). Under higher magnifcation it can be seen that the alveolar structure is retained but the walls are notably thickened and infiltrated by mononuclear cells. The air sacs are free from exudate, but there is a heavy deposit of hyaline material on the surface, which would greatly impede the absorption of oxygen. A similar appearance is found in hyaline membrane disease of neonates and in radiation pneumonitis.(A = air sac, B = alveolar wall, C = hyaline material.)

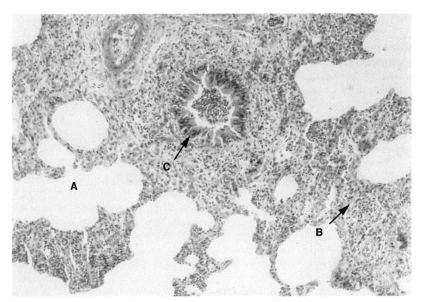

361

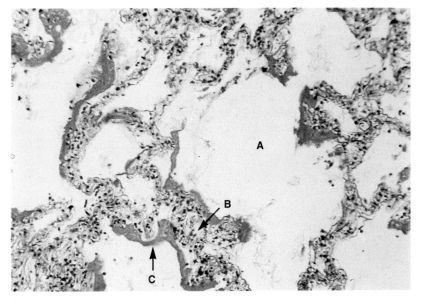

362

Mumps

Mumps is a generalised viral infection with a predilection for the salivary glands, but many other structures may be affected, and inflammation of the testes, pancreas, or central nervous system may be the only manifestation. Subclinical attacks are very common and account for about 30% of all cases of mumps.

Mumps is only moderately infectious, and humans are the only reservoir of infection. The virus is disseminated by infected saliva and gains access through the respiratory passages. Virus may also be found in urine, but there is no evidence that this is important in the spread of mumps.

Myxovirus parotidis possesses haemagglutinin and haemolysin. Filamentous forms are not found. It is a single antigenic entity distinct from other myxoviruses. Mumps virus has two complement-fixing antigens, V (viral antigen), and S (soluble antigen). Following active infection V antibody develops slowly but persists, whereas S antibody appears during the first week of illness, reaches a peak, and then declines.

Virology

363   Normal monkey kidney cell culture.

364   Mumps virus in monkey kidney cells. Mumps virus grows rather more slowly in chick embryo than does influenza virus. It does not have a cytopathogenic effect, but may be detected in the amniotic fluid by agglutination of fowl red blood cells.

Isolation of the virus may be best achieved in cultures of HeLa, human amnion, or monkey kidney cells, in which it produces a cytopathic effect with formation of giant cells and cytoplasmic inclusions. The presence of virus may be shown by haemadsorption with chick, human, guinea-pig, or sheep red blood cells. The supernatant fluid will agglutinate fowl or human red cells.

The diagnosis of mumps is most readily confirmed by complement-fixation tests on paired sera.

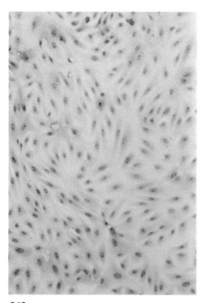

363

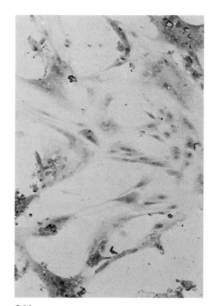

364

Clinical features

365 Parotitis in a child. Mumps is a generalised infection with a wide range of clinical manifestations. Parotitis is common and may be accompanied by inflammation of other structures. Both parotid glands are involved in 70% of patients with parotitis.

The illness begins with fever and malaise, quickly folowed by trismus and pain behind the angle of the jaw. Within 24 hours the parotid gland begins to swell, the hollow behind the angle of the mandible fills, and the swelling extends over the ramus. Confusion sometimes arises with enlarged lymph nodes, but these are usually sited below the parotid gland and the posterior border of the ramus can be sharply defined (see **4**).

366 Parotid papilla in mumps. Redness of the parotid papilla is a helpful early sign. Any fluid discharged from the parotid duct is clear.

367 Parotid papilla in suppurative parotitis. In suppurative parotitis a bead of pus may drip or be expressed from the duct. This form of parotitis is common in debilitated patients but may be found occasionally in previously healthy individuals.

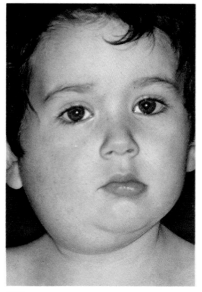

365

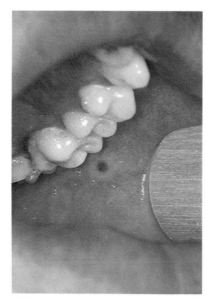

366

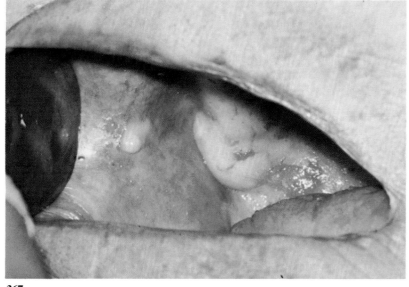

367

368 Parotitis in an adult. Although only 60% of adults are aware of having had an attack of mumps, serological tests show a much higher incidence. The illness tends to be more severe in adults, and the swelling is more painful. Parotitis in the elderly is usually caused by bacterial invasion along the parotid duct.

369 Acute parotitis – oedema of tissues. Swelling of the parotid gland may be accompanied by oedema of the surrounding tissues, which extends into the floor of the mouth and downwards in the neck to the insertion of the deep cervical fascia in the manubrium sterni. This gelatinous oedema is particularly common in coloured people and a sharp tap will produce a jelly-like quivering in the affected tissues.

370 Appearance on recovery. The oedema has subsided and normal appearance has been restored.

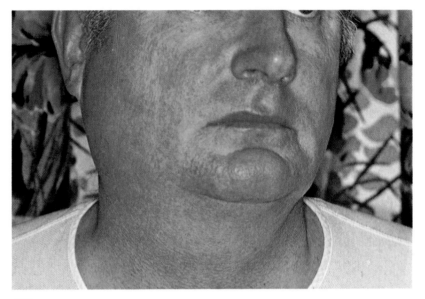

368

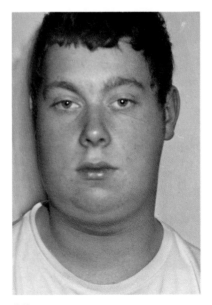

369

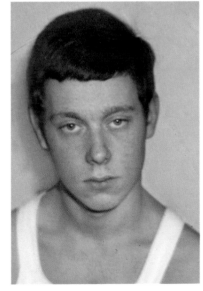

370

309

371 Submaxillary mumps. The submaxillary glands are affected in 10% of patients with mumps. The diagnosis is easy when the parotid glands are also swollen, but otherwise may be exceedingly difficult. A white blood cell count, serum amylase estimation, or complement-fixation tests are helpful in distinguishing submaxillary salivary adenitis from submaxillary lymphadenitis.

372 Orchitis. Mumps orchitis seldom occurs before puberty. It is usually associated with parotitis, but may be the sole manifestation. The incidence varies considerably in different epidemics but averages 20–25% in adolescent and adult males with mumps. It is unilateral in 80% of cases. The testicular swelling may be aggravated by a hydrocele or by oedema of the scrotum.

373 Electrocardiographic changes in mumps. During the acute stage of the illness electrocardiograms are found to be abnormal in 5–15% of cases. The common abnormalities are flattening or inversion of T waves, and depression of the ST segment. The cardiograms return to normal during convalescence. Clinical evidence of myocarditis is rare, but pericarditis may occasionally be detected. Similar electrocardiographic changes are found in many other infections.

The tracings opposite (V_4) were taken from a 10-year-old boy with mumps but no clinical evidence of heart involvement. The first ECG was taken during the acute stage, the second 2 weeks later, and the third after 10 weeks. The myocardial damage has steadily improved.

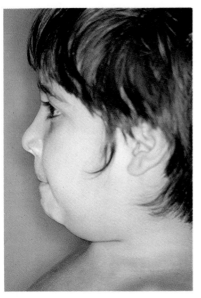

371

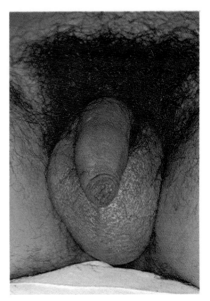

372

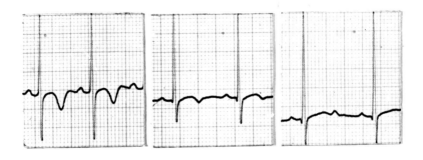

373

Measles

Measles is a highly infectious disease caused by a virus closely related to the larger myxoviruses. Patients are infectious during the acute stage of the illness, and virus is transmitted by the airborne route. There are no carriers, so spread is by direct case-to-case contact. The illness is characterised clinically by a catarrhal prodromal stage, followed by a florid, generalised maculopapular eruption. Damage to the respiratory mucosa facilitates secondary bacterial invasion of the middle ear or lungs. Cerebral disturbance is common and may take several forms. Immunity is life-long.

Virology

374   Electron micrograph of measles virus. Measles virus belongs to the genus *Morbillivirus*, which includes the viruses causing distemper in dogs and rinderpest in cattle. On electron microscopy the virus is roughly circular in outline and measures 120–140 nm in diameter. The outer envelope contains lipid and protein. Haemagglutinin is present, but neuraminidase is lacking. Spikes may be seen radiating from the surface. The nucleocapsid contains RNA and has a helical structure.

375   Normal monkey kidney cells.

376   Measles virus in monkey kidney cells. Primate kidney cells are most effective for primary isolation, but higher concentrations may subsequently be obtained in other tissues. Once isolated, the virus can easily be adapted to continuous cell lines of human origin. It has also been adapted to growth on chick amnion.

The nature of the cytopathic effect varies with the strain of the virus, the type of cell, and the composition of the medium. In primary culture the affected cells form syncytia, but on serial passage the principal change is alteration in the shape of cells from polygonal to spindle. Intranuclear inclusions are a constant finding. Compare with normal monkey kidney cells in **375**.

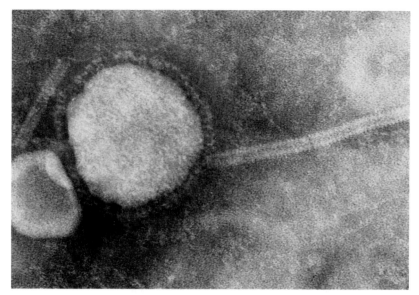

374

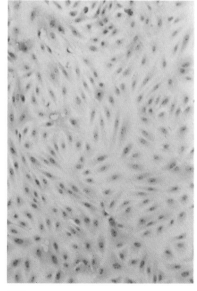

375

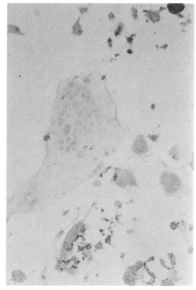

376

Pathology

377   Histology of lung in measles (haematoxylin and eosin stain). During the acute stage of measles the virus may give rise to an interstitial pneumonia resulting in severe respiratory distress. Secondary bacterial invasion of the lungs usually occurs at a later stage, when the rash is fading, and produces a patchy bronchopneumonia.

In the lung section shown here the alveolar pattern has not been disturbed, but the air sacs are packed with mononuclear cells. Very little fibrin is present. Some of the alveoli are lined with hyaline membrane, which can interfere seriously with gaseous exchange. Note the large multinucleated giant cells. (A = air sac with mononuclear cells, B = hyaline material, C = multinucleated giant cell.)

378   Measles pneumonia (histology of lung, red and yellow stain). A large multinucleated giant cell can be seen in the centre of this section. The viral nucleic acid has stained pale pink.

In patients with leukaemia, mucoviscidosis, and Letterer–Siwe disease, where cell-mediated immunity is defective, infection with measles virus may not result in the classical disease but give rise to giant-cell pneumonia, a prolonged and usually fatal illness. (A = giant cell, B = viral nucleic acid.)

379   Histology of appendix (haematoxylin and eosin stain). In the prodromal catarrhal stage of measles, vomiting and diarrhoea are common in young children. The appendix and colon at this stage are infiltrated with mononuclear cells, and giant cells are formed. The congestion of the appendix may be sufficient to cause symptoms of appendicitis. As the rash emerges the multinucleated cells disappear. (A = mucosa, B = lymphoid follicle, C = giant cell.)

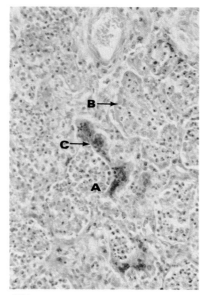

377

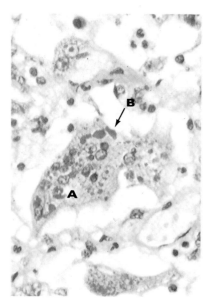

378

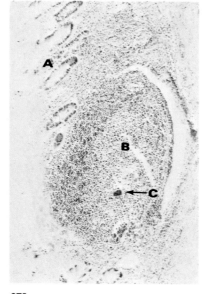

379

380 Appearance of brain in encephalitis. Post-infectious encephalitis usually develops 3–4 days after onset of the rash. The incidence is roughly 1 in 1000 cases. The brain is congested and the essential lesion is demyelination accompanied by microglial proliferation.

Note the severe inflammation of the meninges, the intense congestion of the cortex, and the dilated blood vessels in the white matter.

Clinical features

381 Koplik's spots. Koplik's spots are pathognomonic of measles. They are found on mucous membranes during the prodromal stage and are easily detected on the mucosa of the cheeks opposite the molar teeth, where they resemble coarse grains of salt on the surface of the inflamed membrane. Histologically the spots consist of small necrotic patches in the basal layers of the mucosa with exudation of serum and infiltration by mononuclear cells.

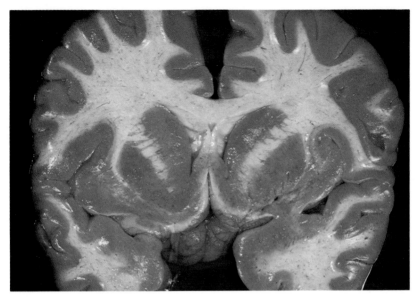

380

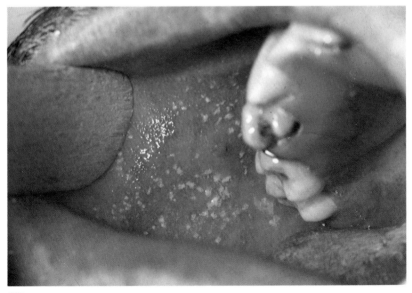

381

382 Koplik's spots and exanthem. Koplik's spots are nearly always present during the early catarrhal stage of measles but disappear as the rash emerges and cannot be seen after the first or second day of the exanthem.

The child in the illustration has a well developed rash on her face, and Koplik's spots are still visible inside her mouth.

383 Appearance of the face in measles. The face has an unmistakable appearance, with suffusion of the conjunctivae, congestion of the buccal cavity, and a dusky-red blotchy rash on the skin.

384 Measles rash on first day. A transient erythematous rash during the prodromal period may be confused with scarlet fever, but careful inspection of the mouth will usually disclose Koplik's spots.

The true rash appears behind the ears and along the hairline, quickly affects the face, and spreads progressively from above downwards. On the first day of the rash the face is heavily covered, but elsewhere the spots are scanty.

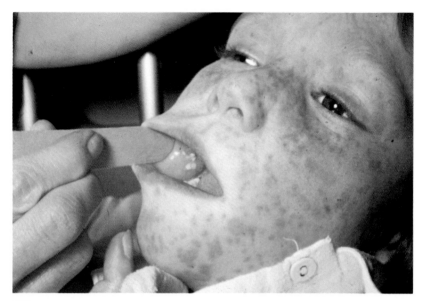

382

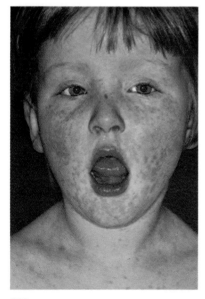

383

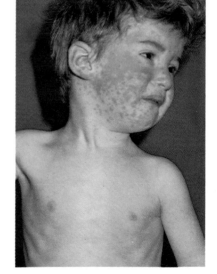

384

385 Close-up of rash. The rash consists of large macules or slightly raised lesions called maculopapules. These run into each other to form irregular blotches.

386 Rash on second day. Large blotches appear on the trunk during the second day of the rash. The evolution of the exanthem from above downwards is helpful in distinguishing it from drug eruptions of a similar nature that seldom follow this course.

387 Rash on third day. By the third day the rash may have become confluent over most of the body, but some discrete spots remain, especially on the limbs.

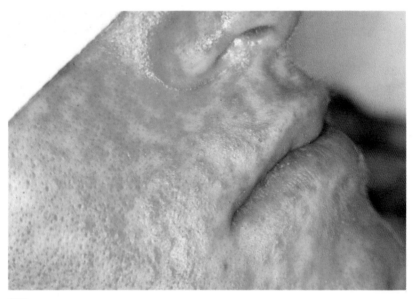

385

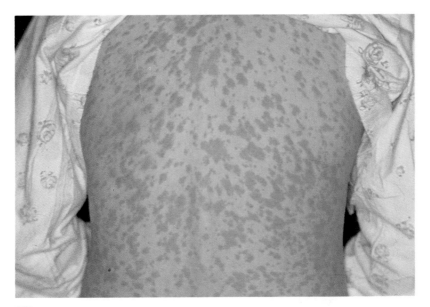

386

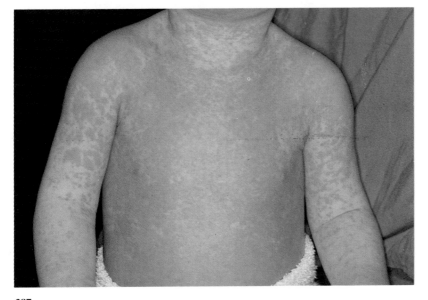

387

388 Measles in a coloured child. Measles may be difficult to diagnose in a dark-skinned patient. Catarrh remains a striking feature and Koplik's spots may be found during the prodromal period.

389 Rash in a coloured child. The erythematous element of the rash is much less conspicuous on a dark skin. The papular component can be thrown into relief by viewing the skin in oblique light.

390 Severe measles. In a severe attack the rash may be confluent over large areas, and fine desquamation may develop. Note the excoriation round the eyes.

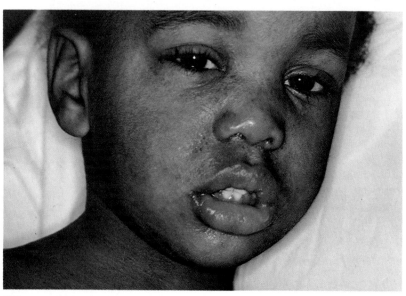

388

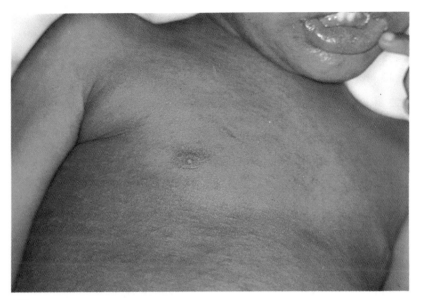

389

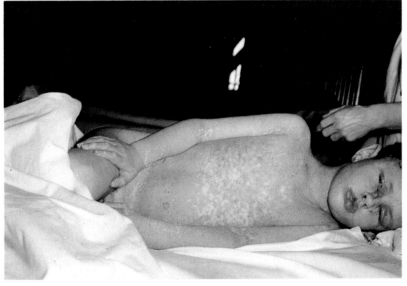

390

391 Staining. The rash fades in the same order as it appears, leaving a brownish pigmentation of the skin called staining. This may be generalised but sometimes has a patchy distribution. In contrast to the original maculopapular rash, the discolouration does not blanch on pressure. Staining may persist for a week or 10 days, then fades without trace.

392 Rash of the secondary stage of syphilis. In secondary syphilis the combination of fever, enlarged lymph nodes and a heavy maculopapular rash (see **200**) may trap the unwary into diagnosing measles. The history and careful clinical examination will usually point to the correct diagnosis, but in doubtful cases it is wise to check the possibility of syphilis by serological tests. The early macular rash of meningocococcal septicaemia, when heavy, may also be confused with measles (see **64**).

393 Erythema multiforme. Erythema multiforme may be mistaken for measles, especially when accompanied by conjunctivitis and stomatitis. The rash in erythema multiforme is pleomorphic, and the individual lesions have a pale centre and a bluish tinge. The rash persists for much longer than that of measles.

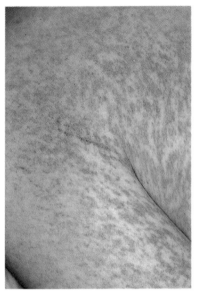

391

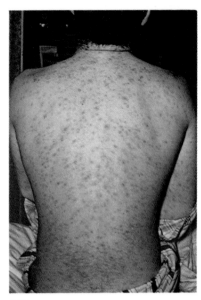

392

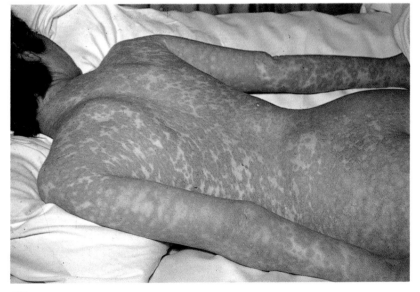

393

Complications

394   Cancrum oris. Children suffering from protein deficiency as a result of malnutrition are exceedingly vulnerable to measles and have a high death rate from gastroenteritis and pneumonia. Necrotic ulceration of the mouth may complicate measles in these children.

395   Secondary bacterial pneumonia. Chest radiograph. Respiratory symptoms during the prodromal and early eruptive stages of measles are caused directly by the virus, which is responsible for catarrhal inflammation of the whole respiratory tract. In young children laryngitis may give rise to alarming symptoms of obstruction, but surgery is seldom required. Acute bronchitis is an integral component of measles and radiographic examination during the eruptive phase may show evidence of viral pneumonitis.

As the rash fades the temperature falls and respiratory distress subsides. Damage to the respiratory mucosa, however, may pave the way for secondary bacterial invasion of the lungs, and the expected defervescence may not take place. Respiratory symptoms increase and radiographic examination may reveal patchy opacities of bronchopneumonia. The white blood cell count may switch from a leucopenia to a polymorphonuclear leucocytosis.

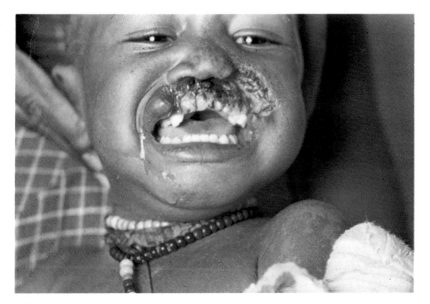

394

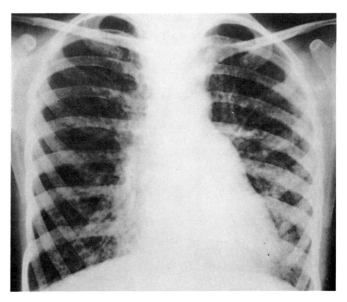

395

327

396 Encephalitis – electroencephalogram. Drowsiness and irritability are constant features with measles, and convulsions are common in young children. Transient abnormalities, with an excess of slow wave patterns, are commonly found in electroencephalograms taken during the acute state of the illness. The EEG quickly returns to normal during convalescence. The incidence of abnormalities is higher in children with febrile convulsions, but is unrelated to the height of the fever. EEG changes are appreciable in encephalitis after measles and may persist after clinical recovery.

The tracings shown here were obtained from a 5-year-old boy who developed mild encephalitis with drowsiness and neck stiffness three days after the onset of the measles rash. Symptoms persisted for 8 days, followed by an uneventful recovery. The EEG returned to normal after 2 weeks.

397 Post-measles encephalitis. Post-infectious encephalitis varies greatly from transient drowsiness to profound coma, resulting in death or severe disability. The child in the illustration has quadriplegia with paralysis in extension caused by this type of encephalitis. The essential lesion is demyelination accompanied by microglial proliferation, possibly the result of damage from an immunological reaction.

Subacute sclerosing panencephalitis is a rare disease that develops several years after an attack of measles. Virus persists in brain tissue after the original attack, causing severe brain damage with proliferation of microglia but minimal demyelination. The illness evolves slowly and inevitably proves fatal within 2 years.

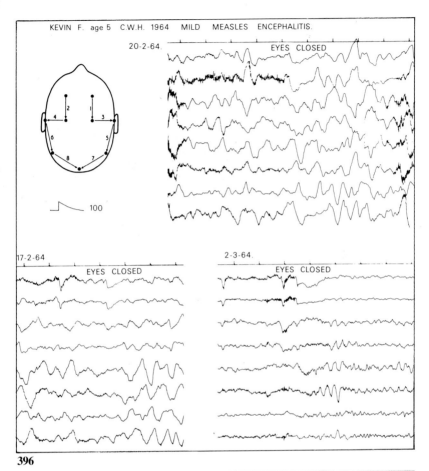

KEVIN F. age 5 C.W.H. 1964 MILD MEASLES ENCEPHALITIS.

20-2-64.   EYES CLOSED

17-2-64.
EYES CLOSED

2-3-64.
EYES CLOSED

396

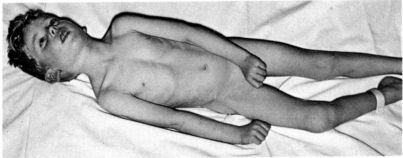

397

Rubella

Rubella is a virus disease with a worldwide distribution. Epidemics occur at irregular intervals of 6–9 years, and the pattern of disease tends to vary from one epidemic to another, suggesting the existence of more than one strain of the virus. In most countries over 80% of the population have developed antibodies against rubella by early adult life.

Postnatal rubella is usually a trivial illness and may occur with or without a rash. Clinical diagnosis is very difficult and often impossible because many other viral infections produce a similar pattern of disease. For accurate diagnosis, antibody tests should be performed on paired sera or specific antibody should be demonstrated in IgM. Virus is present in the throat for at least a week before and after the onset of the rash, and infection is usually transmitted by droplets.

Active infection with rubella during pregnancy results in congenital rubella. The consequences are varied and unpredictable, ranging from fetal death to birth of an infected, but otherwise normal child. The risk to the fetus is greatest in early pregnancy, and the timing of the attack is critical in determining the site of maximal damage. Virus may be shed from the respiratory passages and urine for many months after birth.

Virology

398 Normal rabbit kidney cells (RK13).

399 Rubella virus in RK13 cells. Rubella virus is rounded or ovoid in shape and measures 120–180 nm in diameter. It contains RNA and its infectivity is readily destroyed by ether or chloroform and extremes of pH.

The virus grows on primary and continuous cultures of many mammalian cells and produces subclinical infection in several species of laboratory animal. Vervet monkey kidney cells are widely used for isolating the virus, but there is no cytopathic effect, and activity of rubella virus is recognised by interference with growth of a challenge dose of an enterovirus or by indirect immunofluorescent or immunoperoxidase techniques.

In a line of rabbit kidney cells (RK13) the virus regularly produces a cytopathic effect with focal changes and inclusions within the cytoplasm. Cells, destroyed by the virus, pile up as islets on the uniform culture sheet to form characteristic microfoci.

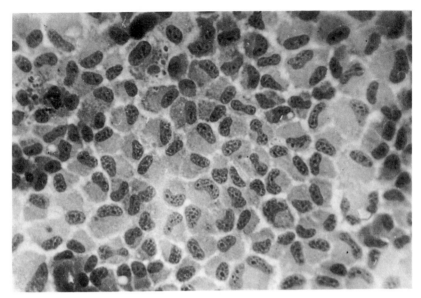

398

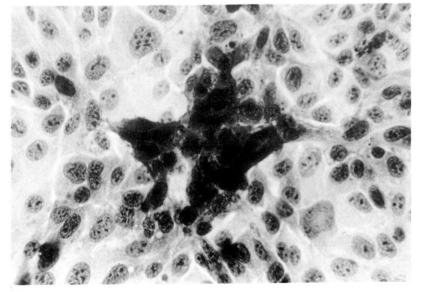

399

Postnatal rubella

400   Throat in postnatal rubella. Rubella acquired after birth is usually a trivial illness and may manifest with or without a rash. The throat may be painful and slightly inflamed, but exudate is seldom present. There is complete absence of coryza, and the buccal cavity is clean and pale. Koplik's spots are never found.

Rubella in young children often occurs without a rash and is indistinguishable from the numerous other viral infections to which they are prone. Such children form an important reservoir of infection for pregnant women.

401   Conjunctivitis in rubella. The conjunctival injection in rubella is not as marked as in measles and there is no discharge from the eyes. The degree of congestion of the conjunctivae and buccal cavity is of value in differentiating rubella from measles and scarlet fever. In rubella the eyes are suffused but there is no congestion of the buccal cavity; in measles both are inflamed; in scarlet fever the buccal cavity is congested but the eyes remain clear.

402   Rubella rash on first day. The rash consists initially of discrete, delicate pink macules, but sometimes maculopapular and haemorrhagic elements may be found. The severity of the rash varies considerably and is easily missed when lesions are sparse.

Similar rashes may be found in many other virus infections, notably echovirus infections. The clinical diagnosis of rubella is most unreliable and less than half the suspected cases are confirmed when antibody tests are performed on paired sera.

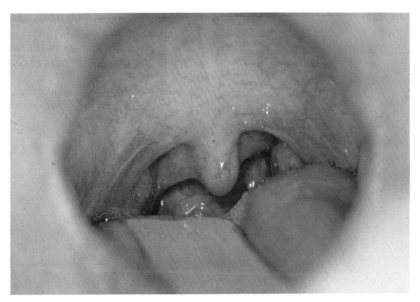

400

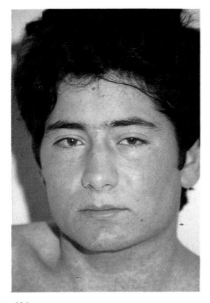

401

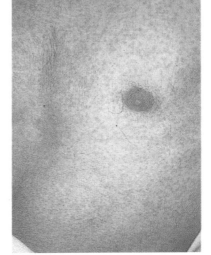

402

403 Rubella versus measles. Although the typical rash of rubella, with its fine pink macules, can easily be distinguished from the blotchy, dusky-red, maculopapular rash of measles, the difference is not always so clear cut. Confusion may arise when the rubella rash has a coarse maculopapular element, but the short duration of the prodromal period and the absence of respiratory catarrh point to the correct diagnosis. When there is doubt, the matter may be settled by demonstrating a four-fold rise in antibody titre between acute and convalescent samples of serum, or by demonstrating rubella-specific antibody in IgM.

404 Rubella rash on second day. The evolution of the rash may be arrested at the macular stage, but more often the individual lesions on the trunk coalesce to produce a pinkish flush, closely resembling the rash of scarlet fever but lacking its punctation.

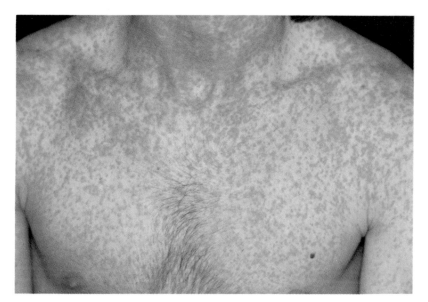

403

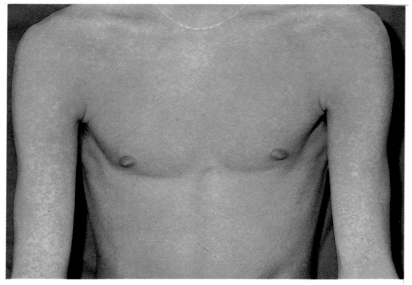

404

405 Rash on thighs – second day. Although the rash on the trunk may become confluent, the macules on the limbs remain discrete, and fresh lesions may appear on the feet. The rash usually fades on the third day and is not followed by staining or desquamation.

406 Purpura in rubella. A purpuric rash, consisting of petechiae and occasional ecchymoses, may occur during the acute state of rubella or in late convalescence after the exanthem has faded. The condition usually resolves spontaneously.

Congenital rubella

407 Congenital rubella – purpuric rash. A purpuric rash is much more common in congenital than in postnatal rubella. The skin haemorrhages may be present at birth or develop within 48 hours. The rash varies greatly in severity and may be accompanied by bleeding from mucosal surfaces. The initial platelet count is usually low, but in surviving infants it returns to normal within one to four months.

The highest incidence of purpura occurs in infants infected during the fourth to eighth week of pregnancy. Mortality is about 30%.

408 Purpura and hepatomegaly. Purpura is commonly associated with other serious defects. Some infants develop pronounced anaemia with erythroid hyperplasia, which may persist for several months. A high proportion have hepatomegaly, splenomegaly, congenital heart disease, and eye defects. Infection is widely disseminated, and virus has been detected in most organs.

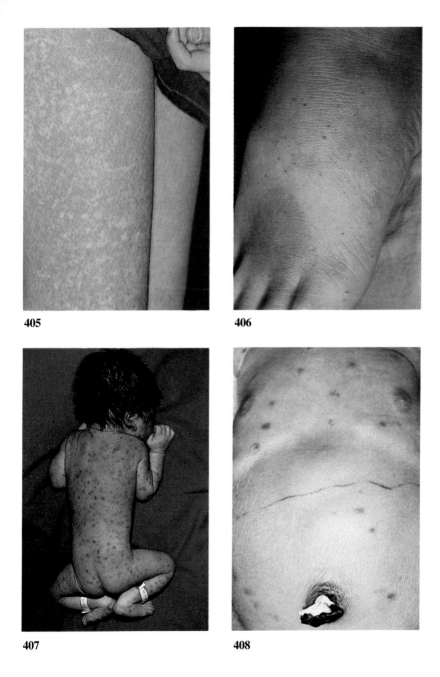

405

406

407

408

337

409 Histology of liver in congenital rubella (haematoxylin and eosin stain). Enlargement of the liver is often present in congenital rubella, but may not be detected until the second or third month of life. The spleen may also be enlarged. Jaundice may appear within a few hours of birth and the serum bilirubin reaches high levels of concentration. Anicteric hepatitis may also occur and serum transaminase concentrations may be raised for several months.

Rubella virus has a cytolytic action, and the local inflammatory reaction is minimal. The liver changes may be diffuse or focal. In the section shown here many liver cells have been destroyed, and the surviving parenchymal cells are swollen and have vacuoles in the cytoplasm. The damaged area has been infiltrated by mononuclear cells.

410 Radiograph of chest – congenital heart disease. Several disabling defects may follow an attack of rubella during the second month of pregnancy when the fetal heart is developing. Patent ductus arteriosus, with or without stenosis of the pulmonary valve or artery, is by far the commonest lesion. Cyanotic heart disease is rare and probably a fortuitous association.

The original 'rubella syndrome' of congenital heart disease, cataracts, and deafness has been extended to include defects of many other organs, as well as general impairment of growth and development.

411 Histology of heart in congenital rubella (haematoxylin and eosin stain). Electrocardiographic evidence of myocardial damage may be found during life. In fatal cases histological examination of the heart shows extensive myocardial necrosis with no inflammatory response. The muscle fibres become swollen and fragmented. In severely affected areas they may be unrecognisable. The nuclei are pleomorphic and pyknotic.

412 Cloudy cornea in congenital rubella. Corneal haze of varying degree may be present at birth, possibly because of oedema in the stromal layers. It can be distinguished from glaucoma because the diameter of the cornea, the depth of the anterior chamber, and the ocular tension are all normal. The cloudiness usually clears progressively during the first few weeks of life.

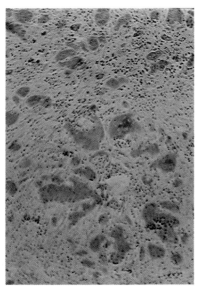

409

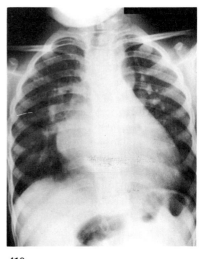

410

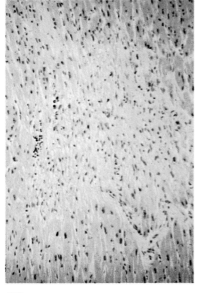

411

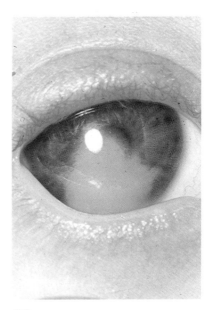

412

413 Glaucoma caused by congenital rubella. Glaucoma is present in 4% of patients with congenital rubella. The cornea is extremely hazy, and its diameter increased. The anterior chamber is deep, and ocular tension is appreciably increased. Following early operation the tension may be restored to normal and the corneal haze clear. Rubella virus has been isolated from aqueous fluid.

414 Cataract in congenital rubella. Spread of virus to the lens during development gives rise to a cataract. When this occurs between the third and fourth week of pregnancy a dense white opacity results, but if infection takes place later, during the sixth or seventh week, the cataract is small and amorphous and may be difficult to detect without ophthalmoscopic examination. Cataracts may be unilateral or bilateral and are often associated with microphthalmos.

Cataract and pigmentary retinopathy, the eye defects most commonly found in congenital rubella, are often associated with deafness and congenital heart disease – 'rubella triad'. Blindness is a serious handicap to a child with bilateral cataracts, especially when combined with deafness, so surgical treatment should not be delayed unduly after the age of 6 months.

415 Radiograph of long bone in congenital rubella. On radiographic examination changes are found in the long bones of a high proportion of infants with congenital rubella. Irregular areas of radiotranslucency are present in the metaphyses of long bones, but there is no evidence of periosteal reaction. These changes begin in early intrauterine life and clear completely within 6–8 weeks from birth. Rubella virus has been isolated from bone.

The abnormal appearance of the metaphysis is caused by defective deposition and calcification of osteoid, probably secondary to a metabolic or nutritional disturbance. The diaphysis is not affected.

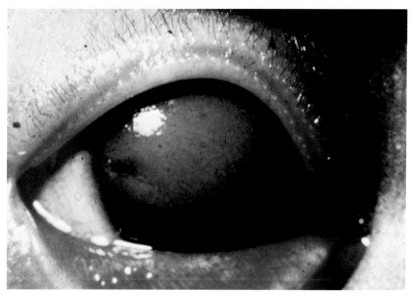

413

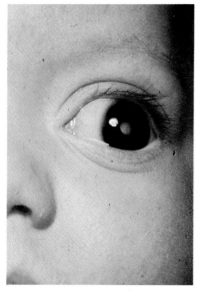

414

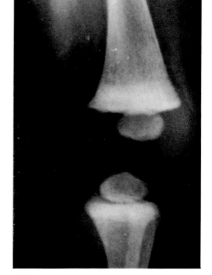

415

Enterovirus infection

The group name, picornaviruses, has been given to large numbers of viruses that are small, resistant to ether, and composed of a core of RNA. The group includes enteroviruses, rhinoviruses and similar viruses of non-human origin. Enteroviruses include the polioviruses, coxsackie viruses and echoviruses. Members of this family do not fall readily into definable categories but grade into each other. Nevertheless, it is convenient to group together those with close affinities.

Enterovirus infection is asymptomatic in 50–80 % of cases, but may cause a mild febrile illness. Systemic invasion may result in more serious illness with infection of the nervous system and other organs. These viruses are responsible for a large variety of clinical syndromes and the same symptom complex can result from infection by a number of them.

Infection is common in young children and is usually symptomless; adult infection, although less common, causes illness more frequently, but is rare in areas with poor standards of hygiene and sanitation, where infection is endemic. In temperate climates enterovirus infections are more prevalent in late summer and autumn; in tropical zones incidence is high throughout the year. Enteroviruses are usually spread by ingestion of faecally contaminated material, although a few serotypes are spread by respiratory droplets. The virus enters the body through the mouth, replicates in the lymphoid tissues of the gastrointestinal tract and is excreted in the faeces. Bloodstream invasion may lead to neurological or other systemic manifestations. Virus is present in the throat and faeces within a few days of infection and up to 7 days before onset of symptoms. It may persist in faeces for as long as 2–3 months.

Because gastrointestinal infection is very common and not necessarily significant, virus isolation from faeces and throat washings should be supported by demonstrating a fourfold rise in specific humoral antibody to confirm a diagnosis of systemic infection. However, isolation of an enterovirus from a normally sterile fluid, such as cerebrospinal or pericardial, is usually relevant. Serological tests alone are impracticable for diagnosis because of the multiplicity of enterovirus types.

416 Electron micrograph of enterovirus. Enterviruses are small spheres with a protein shell and an inner core of RNA. They measure 15–30 nm in diameter. They are very resistant to ether, chloroform, and bile salts. Enteroviruses differ from rhinoviruses by their ability to withstand a pH as low as 3 and heating to 50°C for 1 hour in the presence of molar $MgCl_2$. They have been classified into three serotypes of poliovirus, 24 serotypes of coxsackievirus type A, six serotypes of coxsackievirus type B, and 30 serotypes of echovirus, but it should be stressed that the division is arbitrary, and the separate categories merge into each other.

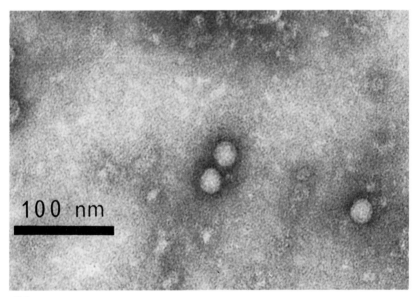

416

417 Normal monkey kidney cells.

418 Poliovirus in monkey kidney cells. All enteroviruses, with the notable exception of some type A coxsackieviruses, grow on monkey kidney cells, producing cytopathic effects. These viruses will also grow on other continuous lines of cells derived from normal and malignant tissues. Some type A coxsackieviruses fail to grow on tissue culture unless specially adapted after primary isolation in suckling mice.

The characteristic cytopathic effect is clearly evident when this illustration is compared with **417**. The uniform cell sheet has been disrupted. The cells are rounded with pyknotic nuclei. At a later stage they separate from the wall of the culture tube.

Exanthematous disease

Echovirus infection

419 Petechial rash in echovirus type 9 infection. In echovirus type 9 infections the rash appears shortly after the onset of the illness and consists of pinkish macules, which fade quickly on the trunk but may persist on the face, where they are more blotchy and have a purplish hue. Sometimes the rash has a petechial character as in this illustration.

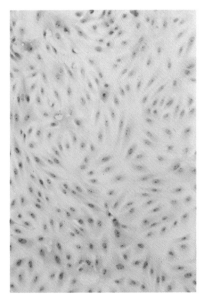

417

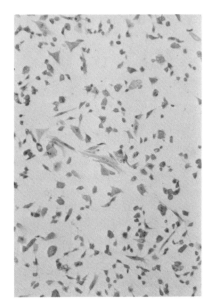

418

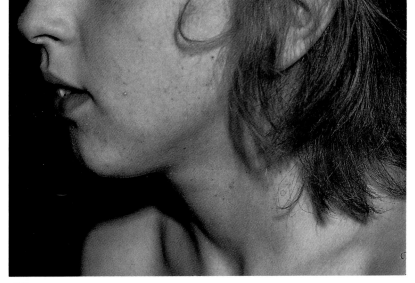

419

420 Rash on trunk – echovirus type 19. The rash on the trunk of the child has a similar appearance, but is less profuse.

As a general rule, it is not possible to determine the type of echovirus from the nature of the rash. Maculopapular, vesicular, petechial and pleomorphic rashes have been described, but it is seldom feasible to recognise a clinical pattern in the absence of an outbreak. Infections with echovirus 16 are characterised by pinkish maculopapular eruptions, which tend to emerge as other symptoms subside.

421 Maculopapular rash on face in echovirus type 19 infection. Aseptic meningitis is the syndrome most commonly associated with echoviruses. Febrile illness with a rash, occurring alone or in conjunction with meningitis, is the next most common manifestation. Paralysis, encephalitis, minor respiratory illness, and diarrhoea have each been linked with echovirus infection.

Maculopapular rashes have been found in infections with echovirus 4, 11, 16, and 19. Such exanthemata may simulate rubella and it may not be possible to arrive at an accurate diagnosis without laboratory tests. A blotchy maculopapular rash is present on the face of this child from whom echovirus type 19 was isolated.

Coxsackievirus infection

422 Maculopapular rash on face in coxsackievirus infection. Maculopapular, petechial, and vesicular eruptions have been described in infections with coxsackieviruses, notably A9, A16, A10, A5, B3, and B5. Other types have been implicated in sporadic cases.

A maculopapular rash is seen on the face of a young girl with a febrile illness caused by a coxsackievirus infection.

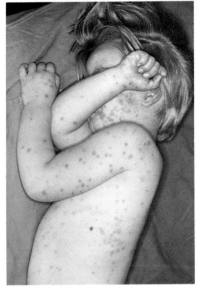

420

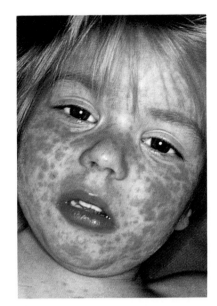

421

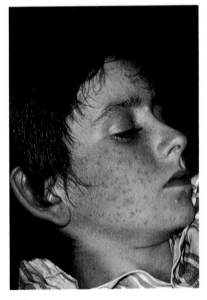

422

Herpangina

423 Herpangina. Herpangina is predominantly a disease of children and is caused by type A coxsackieviruses. It is characterised by an acute onset, with fever, sore throat, and dysphagia. Headache and myalgia are common symptoms, and abdominal pain may add to the distress.

The throat is inflamed, and small discrete vesicles, each surrounded by a band of erythema, may be seen scattered over the palate, fauces and pharynx. The vesicles rupture and leave shallow ulcers which heal within a week. The original vesicles are small, measuring 1–2 mm in diameter, and are replaced by much larger ulcers, measuring up to 5 mm across.

424 Herpes simplex versus herpangina. Herpes simplex may produce similar lesions, but they tend to affect the anterior half of the buccal cavity, whereas herpangina is confined to the posterior.

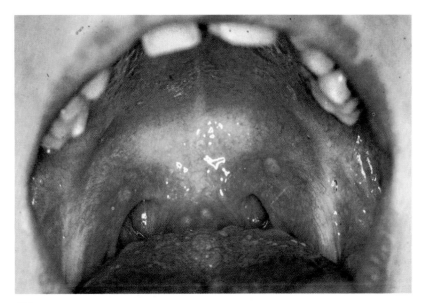

423

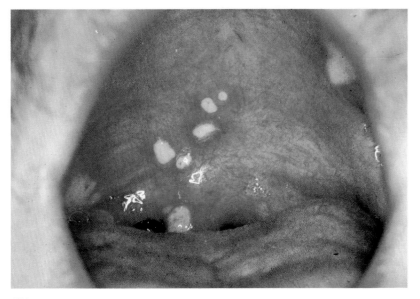

424

349

Hand, foot and mouth disease

425 Hand, foot and mouth disease – vesicles on hand. Hand, foot and mouth disease is a mild illness caused by coxsackieviruses types A16, A10, and A5. Infection occurs in small outbreaks and spreads readily within schools or family groups. After a short incubation period of 3–7 days the illness begins with fever, slight malaise, and a sore mouth. Characteristic lesions appear in the mouth and on the hands and feet. The syndrome occurs more commonly and with more severity in children than in adults.

The lesions on the hands are distributed mainly on the lateral aspects of the fingers but may be found on the palm. The rash is not profuse.

426 Hand, foot and mouth disease – vesicles on finger. The lesions on the skin may consist of bright red macules, small vesicles, thin bullae, or grey ulcers inside a red base.

427 Hand, foot and mouth disease – vesicles on heel. Similar lesions may be found on the feet, particularly on the toes and along the lateral border. Lesions on the feet are seldom seen in children under 3 years of age.

428 Hand, foot and mouth disease – vesicles on toe. The vesicles are superficial and generally heal within a week. There is very little discomfort.

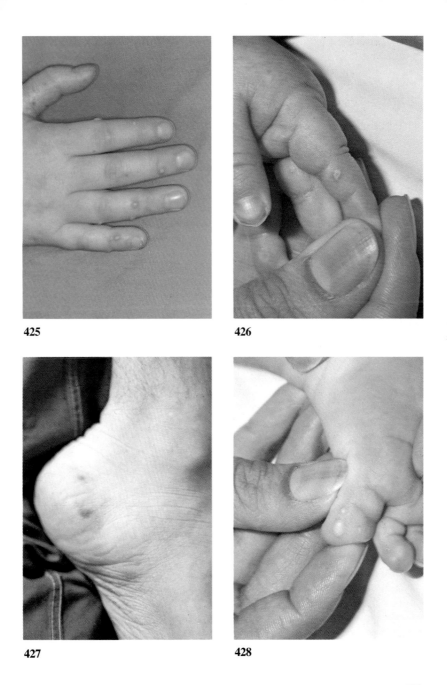

425

426

427

428

429 Hand, foot and mouth disease – lesions in the mouth. The mouth lesions are bright red macules, small vesicles on an erythematous base, or painful, shallow ulcers. They may be found on all parts of the mouth but are seldom seen on the tonsils, and usually only a few lesions are present. The pharynx and the skin round the lips are not affected.

430 Hand, foot and mouth disease – rash on buttocks. A maculopapular rash on the buttocks appears to be part of the syndrome in young children.

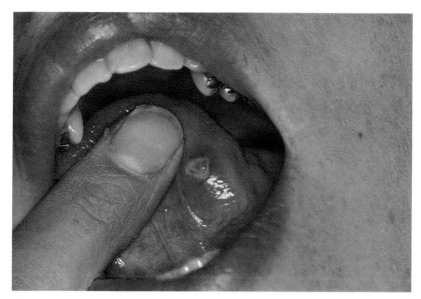

429

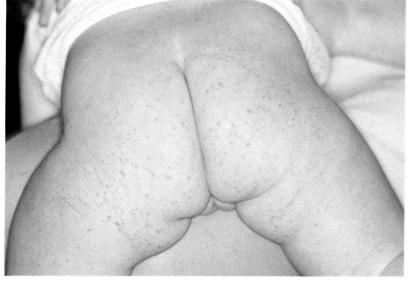

430

353

431 Hand, foot and mouth disease versus gonococcal rash. In adults gono-coccaemia may be accomplished by a vesicular or pustular eruption on the hands that could be mistaken for hand, foot and mouth disease. Mouth lesions are absent and there is usually a history of urethritis or vaginal discharge. Blood cultures and swabs from the skin lesions may grow gonococci (see **184–186**).

432 Hand, foot and mouth disease versus herpes simplex. Herpetic lesions are usually confined to one finger, whereas the rash of hand, foot and mouth disease is more widespread (see **296**).

Roseola infantum

433 Rash on trunk. Roseola infantum, exanthem subitum, or sixth disease, is believed to be caused by a virus infection with an incubation period of 10–15 days. At the onset of illness the young child becomes feverish and may have a convulsion. On examination, the throat is inflamed but there is no exudate. After 3–4 days the fever settles and an erythematous macular rash appears. This persists for 36 hours, then fades. If the child has been given treatment with an antibiotic the rash may be mistaken for drug hypersensitivity. Convulsions are common at onset of illness but other complications are rare.

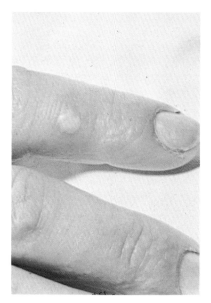

431

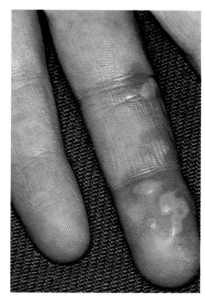

432

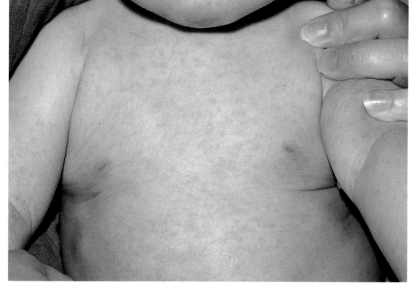

433

Erythema infectiosum (slapped-cheek syndrome)

Erythema infectiosum, also called fifth disease, is a mild infection caused by a parvovirus. In young children the disease follows a benign course; in adults it is less common, though tends to be more severe with a high incidence of arthritis and post-viral debility.

434 Rash on face. There may be a short prodromal period of mild fever with headache, sore throat, and slight gastrointestinal disturbance, before a rash emerges on the face. In many cases the prodrome is absent. The erythema on the face has a blotchy appearance, suggesting the marks of slapped cheeks, and may be associated with circum-oral pallor.

435 Rash on trunk. Either concurrently or within a few days an erythematous rash emerges on the limbs and trunk. It varies considerably in appearance and may be morbilliform, annular, or confluent. The rash often takes on a lacy appearance owing to patches of pallor, and has a notable tendency to come and go over a period of a week or more. Recurrence of the rash may be precipitated by hot baths, exercise or emotional upset. As a rule there are no other findings in children, but adults may have lymphadenopathy and may develop arthritis, especially of the wrists and knees.

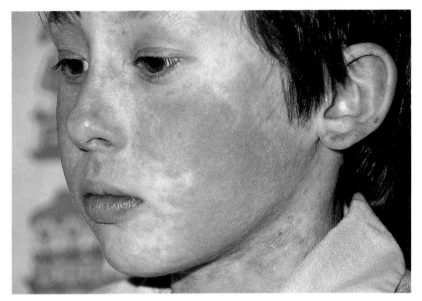

434

435

357

Rabies

Rabies is a viral disease transmitted to humans almost without exception by the bite or saliva of an infected dog. Many other animals may be infected, however, and wildlife populations form the chief reservoir for the disease. Rabies is worldwide in its distribution, with the exception of Australasia and Antarctica. Strict control is possible only on islands such as Great Britain, where control has been effective for many years.

436 Electron micrograph of virus. Rabies virus belongs to a family of single-stranded RNA viruses called rhabdoviruses. The virion measures 75×180 nm and is bullet-shaped, being flat at one end and conical at the other. The surface, except at the flat end, is covered with spikes composed of glycoprotein, which protrude through the surface membrane from the nucleocapsid. This glycoprotein is strongly antigenic and generates neutralising antibody. Virulence of rabies virus appears to be associated with the structure of its glycoprotein.

437 Infected dog bite. The virus usually gains access through a bite from an infected animal and may multiply locally before being transported passively within the axoplasm of nerves to the spinal cord and brain. After further proliferation in the central nervous system the virus spreads peripherally along the same nerve pathways to the tissues of the body. Immunisation with vaccine, after exposure, together with immune serum, has been most successful in preventing rabies. The introduction of vaccines prepared on human diploid cells has virtually eliminated the neurological complications associated with the earlier vaccines.

438 Negri bodies. The early clinical picture may not immediately suggest a diagnosis of rabies, although later the illness is usually characteristic. In the past, the only means of confirming the diagnosis was by the demonstration of Negri bodies in nerve tissue, especially the hippocampus and cerebellum. Negri bodies are sharply defined eosinophilic cytoplasmic inclusions, measuring 2–10 mm and consisting of viral nucleoprotein. They may not always be detected by routine histological staining, and specific staining with fluorescein-labelled rabies antibody may be required. During life the diagnosis can be made by using this type of antibody to stain infected cells from impression smears of the cornea or from skin biopsies.

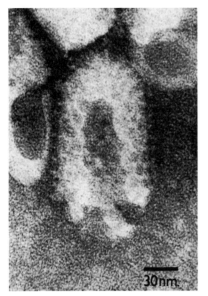

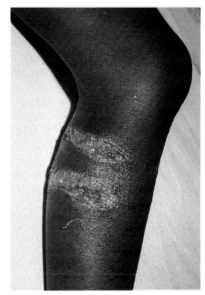

436

437

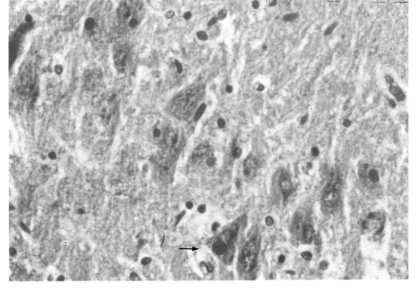

438

439 Hydrophobia. The initial symptoms are headache, loss of appetite, nausea, and vomiting, generally accompanied by mild fever. Some abnormal sensation, such as numbness or tenderness, is a helpful early diagnostic sign. Symptoms of acute anxiety may be present. After 3–4 days the symptoms become progressively worse; the patient is restless and excited and probably hypersensitive to stimuli. Nevertheless, the patient's mind remains quite clear and he or she is able to answer questions in an intelligent manner. The characteristic feature of hydrophobia may then develop. On attempting to drink (or even considering it) the muscles of swallowing and respiration go into sudden spasm so that any fluid is violently ejected and the head thrown back. Spasms, however, may be induced by a variety of stimuli and may also occur spontaneously as part of a generalised hyperactive state interspersed by periods of calm. Life may be terminated abruptly by respiratory obstruction or cardiac arrest, or gradually by progressive paralysis.

440 'Dumb' rabies. In perhaps 20% of patients hyperactivity is absent and paralysis is predominant, as seen in this child with the expressionless face of 'dumb' rabies. The boy is drooling saliva because of paralysis of the muscles of swallowing.

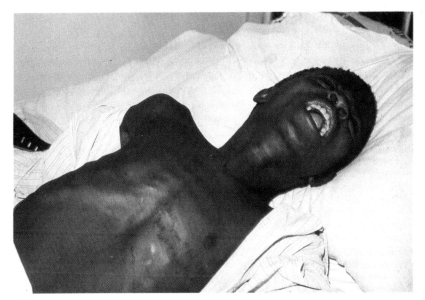

439

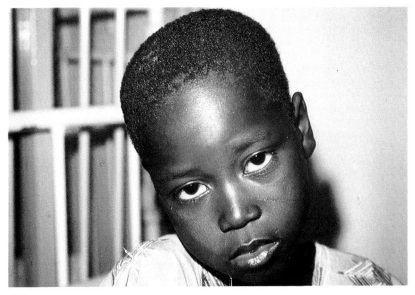

440

Poxvirus infections

The poxviruses are the largest and most complex of true viruses, causing pox infections in many mammals and birds, myxomatosis in rabbits, and molluscum contagiosum in humans. The viruses are oval when hydrated, and brick-shaped when dried for electron microscopy. They contain DNA and most have an uneven, mulberry-like surface because of the presence of threads in the surface structure. Sensitivity to ether varies within the group. Multiplication appears to take place entirely within the cytoplasm of the host cell. Viral particles may be liberated when the host cell disintegrates or may spread directly to contiguous cells.

Orthopoxviruses of humans are no longer important since the eradication of smallpox in 1979. A few cases of clinical smallpox have been recognised in people living on the edges of the tropical rain forests in Africa, but there is little evidence of case-to-case transmission. The disease has been designated monkeypox, and the virus is closely related to, but distinct from, smallpox virus. Parapoxviruses are responsible for such human diseases as orf and paravaccinia (milkers' nodes).

Orf (contagious pustular dermatitis)

441 Orf – electron micrograph of virus. The viruses of orf and paravaccinia have a similar morphology to the poxviruses of the variola group. Orf virus on electron microscopy measures 252 × 158 nm and has a coiled or woven appearance. It does not produce lesions on chick embryo but can be grown in a variety of tissue cultures, including human amnion cells.

442 Orf – infected sheep. Contagious pustular dermatitis is a disease of sheep and goats that occasionally spreads to humans. It is particularly prevalent in lambs and kids. In animals the infection manifests with a papulovesicular eruption on the lips and surrounding skin, but may affect non-wool-bearing areas of skin elsewhere. The virus persists in the soil of an affected pasture for some months, and animals probably become infected while grazing. Infection may spread by direct contact to shepherds or butchers handling infected lambs.

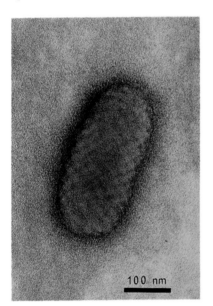

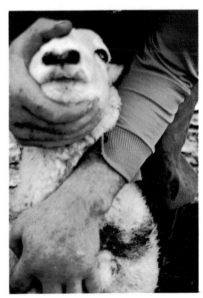

441   **442**

443 Orf – human infection. A lesion may occasionally develop on the face. Although unsightly and slow to heal, it does not usually leave a scar. Virus may be recovered from the lesion by inoculating fluid into tissue culture, or into the scarified skin of a sheep.

444 and 445 Orf – lesions on forearm and hand. In most patients a single papule appears on the skin of the hand, wrist, or forearm and slowly develops into a large, flat vesicle or bulla, which may be haemorrhagic. The surrounding tissues are indurated and inflamed, but the lesion is remarkably free from pain. There is no constitutional disturbance.

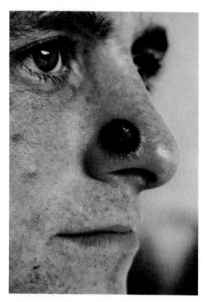

443

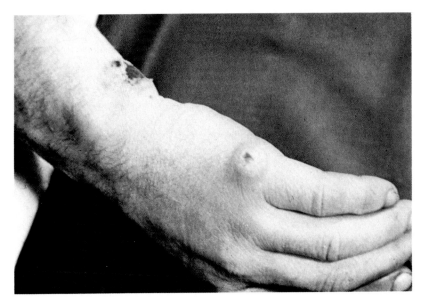

444

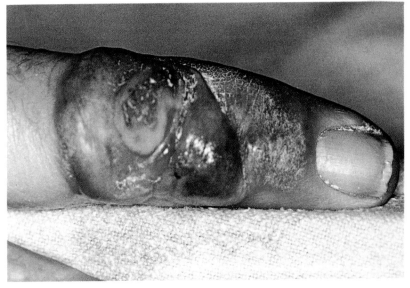

445

Milkers' nodes (paravaccinia)

446 Milkers' nodes – rash on hands. This condition is distinct from cowpox and orf. The virus responsible is closely related to that of orf. It cannot be propagated on chick embryo but can be cultured serially in bovine cells. Human infection is acquired from milking infected cows.

Papular lesions appear on the fingers or hands and increase slowly in size over a period of 1–2 weeks. The nodules are bluish-red in colour and painless. Vesiculation does not occur. The lesions heal without forming a scar. Fever is usually absent, but there may be severe allergic rashes.

447 Milkers' nodes – allergic rash. Nodular lesions are present on the swollen hands, and there is an allergic rash on the face and neck. Note the absence of toxaemia. The regional lymph nodes are seldom enlarged.

Molluscum contagiosum

Molluscum contagiosum is a worldwide human infection caused by an unclassified poxvirus. Infection is transmitted by direct contact or by fomites. Any age group may be affected.

448 Electron micrograph of virus. The virus contains DNA and measures roughly 300×220 nm. It causes a benign infection of the human epidermis and may be found in high concentration in the superficial epithelial cells, where it causes ballooning degeneration and the formation of large hyaline, acidophilic, granular, intracytoplasmic inclusions (molluscum bodies). These contain virus particles similar in appearance to those of orf. With negative staining, the particles resemble balls of yarn on electron microscopy. The virus has not been propagated serially in tissue culture, and no serological tests are available.

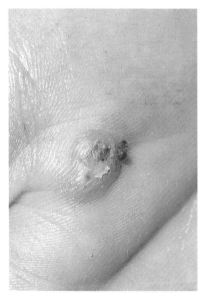

446

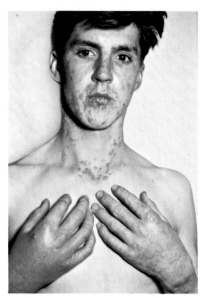

447

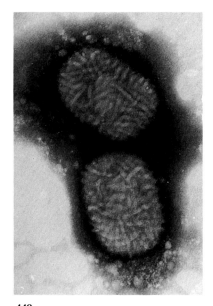

448

449   Skin lesions. The number of lesions varies from one patient to another; any part of the body may be affected except the palms and soles. The lesion begins as a small, firm, shiny, pearly nodule measuring 1–5 mm in diameter.

450   Skin lesions. These slowly enlarge and become umbilicated. Caseous material may be discharged or expressed from the lesions. After a few months the lesions spontaneously regress and heal without scarring.

451   Penile lesions. There is increasing evidence that molluscum contagiosum may be transmitted sexually.

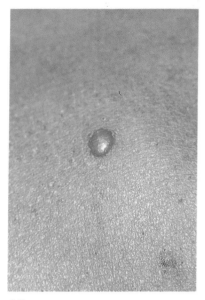

449

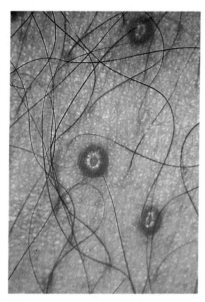

450

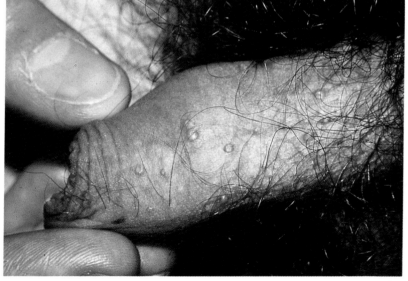

451

369

PROTOZOAL INFECTIONS
Amoebiasis

Amoebiasis is infection with the protozoan parasite *Entamoeba histolytica*. Man is the only host, and infection is usually transmitted by water. The parasite exists in two forms: the vegetative form, capable of division but sensitive to the outside environment; and the cyst, which is incapable of division but is resistant to the environment. Under certain circumstances, not properly understood, the vegetative form may become invasive, penetrating the mucosa of the large bowel and replicating in the submucosa to produce symptoms. In a small proportion of infected individuals amoebae may reach the liver or other organs, replicate, and produce localising symptoms.

452 *Entamoeba histolytica* **cyst.** Diagnosis of amoebiasis is most often made by finding cysts in the stool, usually in an asymptomatic person. The amoebic cyst measures more than 10 μm in diameter, and four nuclei can usually be identified, distinguishing it from the cyst of the non-pathogenic *E. coli* with eight nuclei.

453 *Entamoeba histolytica* **trophozoite.** The trophozoite is not found in the stool unless the patient is asymptomatic; diarrhoea with or without blood, absence of abdominal pain, and lack of constitutional upset are characteristic features. On microscopy the trophozoite, measuring 20–30 μm, is motile and contains ingested erythrocytes. It moves in a characteristic manner with protrusion of a pseudopod, into which the cytoplasm and any ingested red blood cells flow, like a 'bag of marbles' rolling along. The stool is remarkably lacking in inflammatory cells, thereby distinguishing amoebic from bacillary dystentery.

454 Appearance of large bowel. In the submucosa of the large bowel amoebic trophozoites multiply and cause tissue necrosis. This produces the undermined ulcer seen on sigmoidoscopy. Only occasionally do the amoebae penetrate more deeply into the bowel wall and cause perforation. (A = amoeba.)

At necroscopy the bowel may be ulcerated from end to end with multiple perforations. The wall may be extremely friable, with the consistency of wet blotting paper. Such extensive ulceration causes death, especially in the elderly, debilitated, and malnourished.

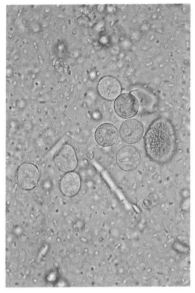

452

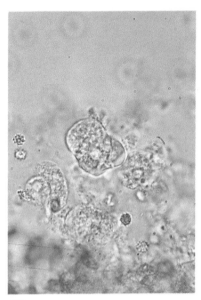

453

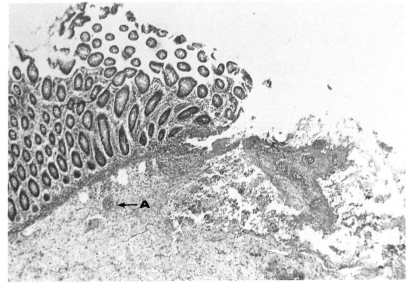

454

455   Liver abscess – ultrasonography. Ultrasonography of the liver confirms the presence of a cavity and distinguishes between an abscess and a cyst. Amoebic abscesses are most commonly found in the right lobe of the liver and may appear multiple on examination. The size and exact location of the abscess may be determined from the scan. (A = abscess.)

456   Liver aspiration. Aspiration was the only method of diagnosis before the invention of scanning. If amoebic material was encountered then aspiration continued as part of treatment; this has now been replaced by chemotherapy. When rupture of an abscess seems imminent or when the response to chemotherapy is slow, aspiration may, however, be beneficial. In parts of the world where scanning and serological tests are not available aspiration is still important for diagnosis and treatment.

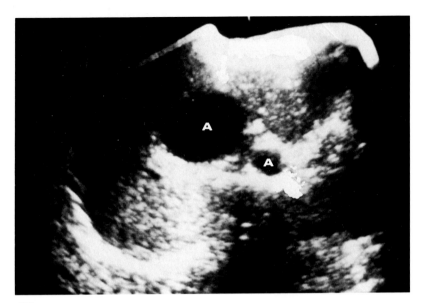

455

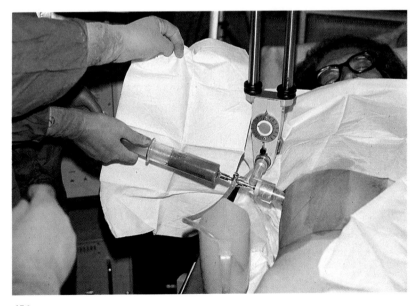

456

457 Liver aspirate. The material aspirated from an amoebic liver abscess has a characteristic appearance and smell. Although described as 'anchovy sauce', the material often has a more reddish tinge. It is not pus in the strict sense of the term, as neutrophils are not present; it consists of necrotic liver tissue, the result of proteolytic enzymes of the trophozoite. The smell of the aspirate is not unpleasant, and culture yields no bacterial growth. Secondary bacterial infection in an amoebic abscess is rare.

458 Amoebiasis of skin. This was a serious complication in the days before effective treatment. It occurred at the site of rupture of an amoebic abscess or in the perineum of debilitated patients with amoebic colitis. Here a misdiagnosed empyema has been drained surgically; the correct diagnosis was liver abscess, which had ruptured through the diaphragm into the pleural cavity.

459 Radiograph of chest. Radiographic examination of the chest may suggest amoebic liver abscess. The radiological features are elevation of the diaphragm, a small pleural effusion, and some linear collapse at the right base. On screening there is reduced or paradoxical movement of the right hemidiaphragm.

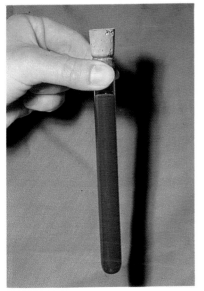

457

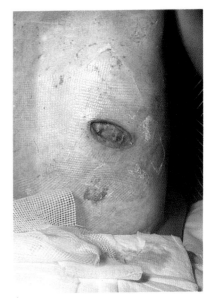

458

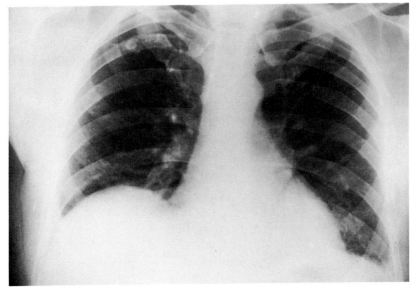

459

375

Malaria

Malaria is caused by protozoan parasites of the genus *Plasmodium* transmitted to man by the bite of female anopheline mosquitoes. Malarial infections are confined to man, who is the intermediate host. The definitive host is the mosquito, in which the sexual forms of the parasites are found. Malaria is almost entirely restricted to the tropics and subtropics; occasionally, however, an infected mosquito may be transported to a non-endemic area and infect man, or an infected person from an endemic area may be the source of infection for a mosquito in a temperate part of the world.

460   Liver schizont. Sporozoites inoculated by the biting mosquito spend a short time in the peripheral blood before localising in the liver. Depending on the species of parasite, the products of the liver schizont are released early or late into the peripheral blood, where they parasitise erythrocytes. The parasites of malignant tertian or falciparum malaria and those of quartan malaria are released early, whereas those of vivax and ovale may be released weeks, months, or even years later.

461   *Plasmodium falciparum* – small rings. The parasite of malignant tertian malaria appears within peripheral erythrocytes as small rings or merozoites. More than one parasite may be seen within a single red blood cell, and the parasitaemia (proportion of red blood cells parasitised) may even be as high as 20%. Further development of the parasite takes place in deep visceral rather than surface vessels.

462   *Plasmodium falciparum* – gametocytes. These sexual forms of the parasite appear in the peripheral blood days or weeks after the asexual forms are first seen and are infectious for mosquitoes. Those of *P. falciparum* are characteristically crescent-shaped.

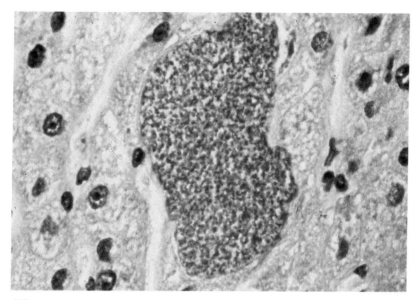

460

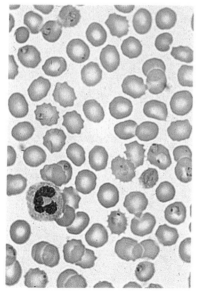

461

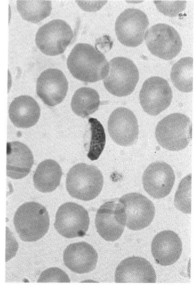

462

463 *Plasmodium vivax*. This species is readily recognised in peripheral blood films, as it fills and enlarges the invaded erythrocyte. Note the characteristic Schüffner's dots. Parasitaemia is seldom greater than 1%, and gametocytes are rarely seen.

464 *Plasmodium ovale*. *P. ovale*, seen in peripheral blood films, is similar to *P. vivax*, but the filled red blood cells tend to be oval and have a somewhat crenated surface. Gametocytes are rarely seen.

465 *Plasmodium malariae*. The parasite of quartan malaria produces febrile paroxysms within a 72-hour periodicity and generally gives a low parasitaemia. Recrudescences resulting from the persistence of blood forms, rather than liver forms, may occur years after the intial infection. The 'band' form seen here is characteristic of *P. malariae*.

466 Nephrotic syndrome. The nephrotic syndrome is a complication of malaria, especially in children infected with *P. malariae*. It differs from the nephrotic syndrome of children in temperate climates in that it occurs at a later age (3–5 years), responds less well to corticosteroids, and has a worse prognosis. Furthermore, it does not respond to antimalarial treatment.

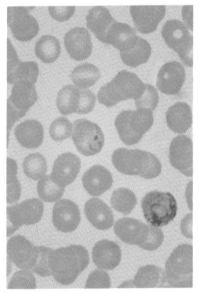

463

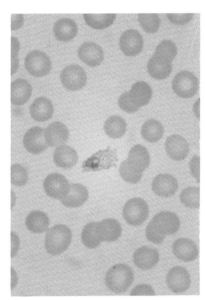

464

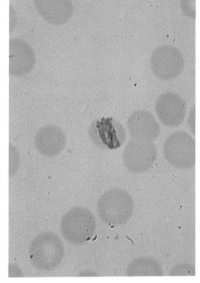

465

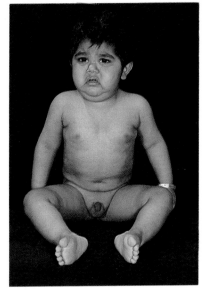

466

467 Jaundice. Fever, rigors and sweating are usually the only abnormal physical findings in an attack of malaria. In falciparum infections, which are responsible for complicated malaria, there may be other signs, including jaundice. This is caused partly by haemolysis and partly by liver damage. When jaundice is pronounced it is often associated with other features of complicated malaria, including cerebral symptoms, renal failure and haemorrhage.

468 Haemorrhage. Thrombocytopenia is common is falciparum malaria but is usually not severe enough to produce bleeding. Occasionally, however, subconjunctival haemorrhage may occur.

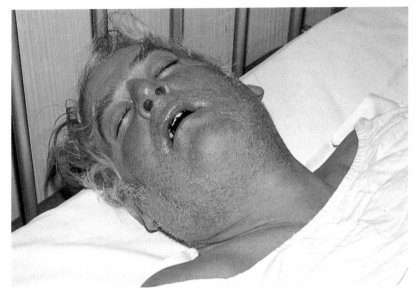

467

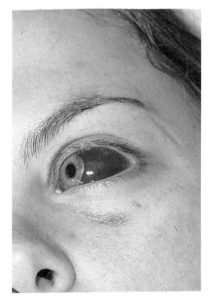

468

469 Histology – cerebral malaria. Only falciparum malaria is fatal. Deterioration may be sudden and can occur even when the patient is taking anti-malarial drugs by mouth. Death is due to the effects of occlusion of visceral vessels packed with parasitised erythrocytes. Cerebral malaria is a manifestation of such occlusion. In the section of brain shown here there is pigment, and the erythrocytes contain dividing parasites (schizonts).

470 Histology – liver. Malarial pigment is prominent in liver sections from fatal cases and in liver biopsy samples from patients living in endemic areas. (A = pigment.)

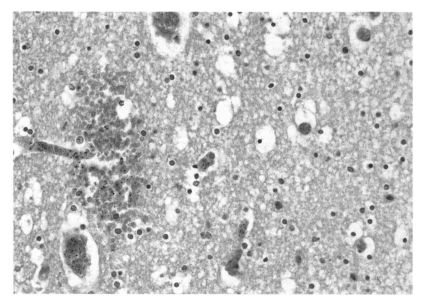

469

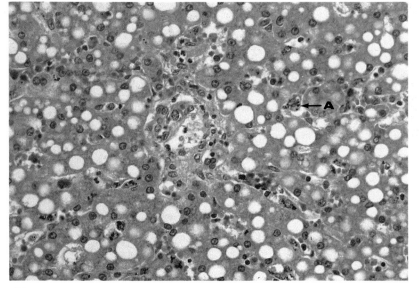

470

383

Toxoplasmosis

Infection with the protozoon *Toxoplasma gondii* is widespread in birds and many mammals, including humans. The incidence in the human population varies considerably throughout the world, and is particularly high in Central America and France. Although human infection is common, clinical disease is rare. It is a frequent manifestation of AIDS, particularly in Africa, and commonly involves the nervous system. During pregnancy, maternal toxoplasmosis spreads readily to the fetus causing death, or serious damage to the eyes or brain. Congenital infection is present in about 40% of infants born to mothers primarily infected during pregnancy. The risk of transmission is lowest in early pregnancy but results in the most severe disease. Most infected infants develop clinical disease.

In acquired toxoplasmosis the common pattern of disease is benign lymphadenitis closely resembling the glandular variety of acute infectious mononucleosis. Examination of the blood may show a lymphocytosis with atypical cells, but the Paul–Bunnell test is invariably negative. The main features of the illness are fatigue and slight lymphatic enlargement, which may be generalised or confined to one region. Convalescence is protracted, but recovery is complete. Toxoplasmosis may occasionally cause encephalitis or fatal generalised disease. The diagnosis is established by detecting humoral antibodies by the Sabin–Feldman dye test, passive haemagglutination or fluorescent methods, the last permitting differentiation of IgM and IgG responses.

- Acute infection: fluorescent (IgM) and dye tests become positive early; passive haemagglutination antibodies appear later; rising titre should be demonstrable.
- Subclinical infection: antibody detectable in low titre (up to 200 i.u.).
- Chronic focal infection (e.g. ocular toxoplasmosis): antibody titres indistinguishable from subclinical infection; IgM response not demonstrable.

Isolation from blood or body fluids by culture in eggs or inoculation of mice is possible but serological diagnosis is more common. Trophozoites or cysts may occasionally be demonstrated histologically in biopsy material.

The toxoplasma exists in three main forms: trophozoite, tissue cyst, and faecal cyst. The trophozoite, or free form, spreads within the host, causing disease. As immunity develops the free forms are destroyed and the parasite enters a cystic phase in the tissues of the eye, central nervous system, and skeletal muscles. These cysts contain zoites and may persist for many years without provoking a host reaction. The sexual cycle takes place in the cat, which is probably infected by eating birds and small rodents; toxoplasmas develop in the gastrointestinal mucosa, forming long-lived faecal oocysts.

The cat is the definitive host, and excretes oocysts in its stools. Infection is widespread in food animals, such as sheep, pigs, goats and cattle. Humans are infected by eating raw or undercooked infected meat, by eating vegetables contaminated with infected soil, or by ingestion of oocysts excreted in cat faeces. Water-borne and milk-borne (goat) outbreaks have been described.

Organism

471 Trophozoites within cytoplasm of host cell (Leishman's stain).
Trophozoites may be found within the cytoplasm of any nucleated cell but are particularly common in cells of the reticuloendothelial system. They are crescent- or pear-shaped with rounded or pointed ends. With Leishman's stain the cytoplasm of the trophozoite is blue and contains a rounded red-stained mass of chromatin, the nucleus. The sizes can be gauged relative to the faintly outlined red blood cells. Reproduction is asexual by longitudinal binary division. Eventually an intracellular colony (pseudocyst) of 16–32 trophozoites is formed.

472 Trophozoites released from cell (Leishman's stain). The host cell ruptures, releasing the trophozoites, which spread throughout the body, invading and multiplying within cells of the reticuloendothelial system until immunity develops, and the free forms are destroyed.

473 Tissue cyst in cerebellum (haematoxylin and eosin stain). As immunity rises cysts form, and the parasite enters another phase of its cycle. These cysts are separated from the host tissues by a tough elastic membrane and do not provoke an inflammatory reaction unless they leak. The young cyst is small and contains only two zoites, which resemble small trophozoites, but the cyst gradually grows as the zoites multiply until it may eventually reach 100 μm in diameter and contain many thousands of zoites.

Tissue cysts are scanty, and many tissue sections may be examined before one is found. Shrinkage during fixation has caused the unstained halo round this cyst in the cerebellum. (Arrow = cyst.)

Pathology

474 Section of infected lymph node showing active germinal centres (haematoxylin and eosin stain). The histological appearance of an infected lymph node is not pathognomonic, and parasitic cysts are seldom found. The lesion is a non-necrotising granuloma with numerous small clusters of large epithelioid macrophages scattered amongst lymphoid tissue. There are no giant cells. A similar appearance is found in early tuberculosis and in sarcoidosis. (Arrow = large epithelioid macrophages.)

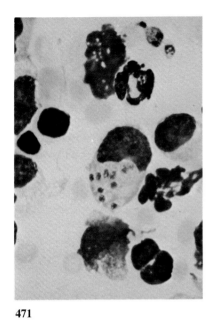

471

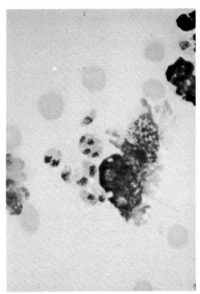

472

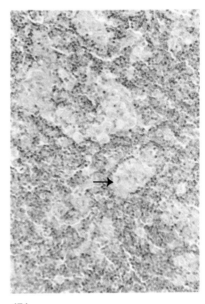

473

474

Clinical features

475 Acute choroidoretinitis.

476 Chronic choroidoretinitis. Clinical or subclinical infection during pregnancy may result in invasion of the fetus by trophozoites. The extent of the damage depends on the age of the fetus and the virulence of the strain of toxoplasma. In early pregnancy infection may cause abortion, but in the later stages evidence of damage may not appear for several weeks after birth. The reticuloendothelial system and muscles are heavily infected initially, but ultimately the parasite tends to localise in the central nervous system, where it may cause severe and lasting damage. The classic triad of hydrocephalus, cerebral calcification, and choroidoretinitis is found in 60% of cases.

Choroidoretinitis is a common manifestation of congenital toxoplasmosis and may be present at birth or develop a few weeks later. In most patients both eyes are affected. Although the eye changes are usually confined to the choroid and retina, adjacent structures may be affected and the eye grossly damaged. When severe, the defect will be obvious shortly after birth. In such cases a white 'reflex' is present, and it may not be possible to inspect the fundus. When infection is less severe it may be overlooked until attention is drawn to the eye by the presence of squinting and nystagmus. Changes in the fundi may be discovered on routine examination of schoolchildren with defective vision. Occasionally older children and adults have acute exacerbations accompanied by haziness of the vitreous and diminished visual acuity.

Once the acute stage has subsided the necrotic tissue is absorbed, leaving an avascular scar through which the sclera often shows. These scars vary in size and may be multiple. They are surrounded by black choroidal pigment.

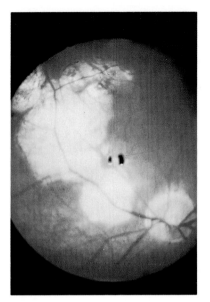

475

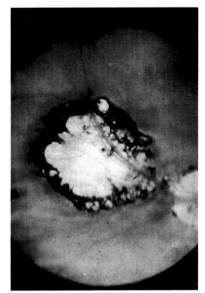

476

477 Hydrocephalus. Cerebral damage is common but may be difficult to recognise during the first few months of life. In the average attack mental retardation is usually present, often accompanied by epilepsy. The cerebrospinal fluid is xanthochromic with increased protein and cells, predominantly mononuclear.

Inflammatory foci with areas of necrosis are scattered throughout the brain and spinal cord but are particularly numerous in the subependymal layer of tissue in the walls of the lateral ventricles. Necrotic fragments may be shed into the ventricles and block the aqueduct, or acute inflammatory oedema may compress the walls of the aqueduct, leading in both cases to obstructive hydrocephalus.

Destruction of brain tissue in the fetus may be so extensive that the brain is shrivelled, and the greater part of the cranial cavity filled with yellow cerebrospinal fluid. 'Pseudocysts' may be present within the areas of necrosis and are a diagostic feature. Painstaking search may occasionally reveal trophozoites lying free in the brain, but they can be detected more readily by inoculating cerebrospinal fluid into young mice.

478 Radiograph of skull showing intracranial calcification. During healing, calcium salts are deposited in the necrotic tissue and may be detected by radiographic examination. Calcification is sometimes present at birth but may be delayed for several months.

On radiographic examination linear streaks may be found parallel to the walls of the lateral ventricles and irregular opacities detected in the subcortex and basal ganglia. It should be appreciated, however, that only 50% of children aged under 1 year with cerebral calcification or choroidoretinitis have toxoplasmosis.

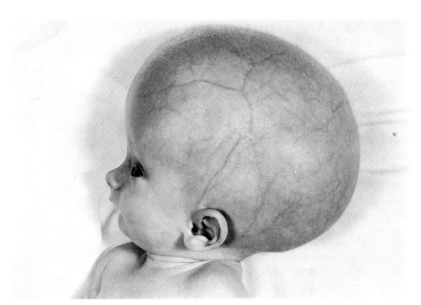

477

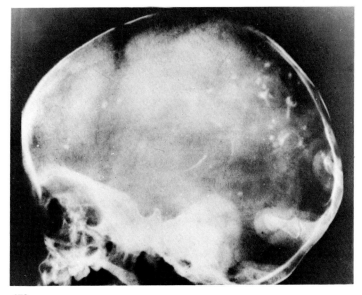

478

MISCELLANEOUS CONDITIONS
Mycoplasma infection

Mycoplasmas, formerly known as pleuropneumonia-like organisms (PPLO), are very small parasitic or saprophytic micro-organisms that are widely distributed in nature. They are responsible for respiratory disease in humans and many animals. *Mycoplasma pneumoniae* (Eaton's agent) has been incriminated as a cause of respiratory illness in humans, while *Mycoplasma hominis* type 1 has come under suspicion as a possible cause of non-specific urethritis and other genital tract infections. Many species are found as commensals in the mouth and genital tract of humans and animals.

Organism

479 Mycoplasma colonies on agar medium. Mycoplasmas are very small pleomorphic organisms, varying in diameter from 0.125 to 0.3 µm. They contain both DNA and RNA but lack a rigid cell wall. Most species will grow aerobically on a cell-free serum-enriched medium but some require additional carbon dioxide. Growth begins with a granule (elementary corpuscle) that enlarges and then divides by multiple fission into fresh granules or filaments. Granules may remain attached to the parent cell, so many different shapes may arise. On solid agar medium the granules are drawn by capillary action into the interstices of the gel and then grow upwards to the surface where a thin layer spreads outwards from the centre of the colony in the film of water on the surface of the agar. The heaped-up, granular centre surrounded by the thin transparent border produces the typical 'fried egg' appearance. The colonies grow slowly but are visible to the naked eye after seven to 12 days. The morphology of the colony varies with the species. Specific antisera labelled with fluorescein can be used to stain the colonies for identification.

480 Beta-haemolysis caused by *M. pneumoniae*. Some species of mycoplasma produce lysis of sheep or guinea-pig red blood cells. The haemolysis may be of α or β type and extends for 2–5 mm around the colonies. Fermentation of sugars can be used to distinguish *M. pneumoniae* from commensal strains found in humans. Each species of mycoplasma appears to be antigenically distinct.

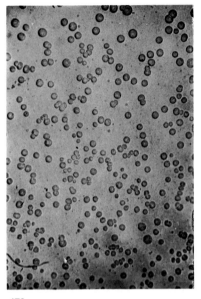

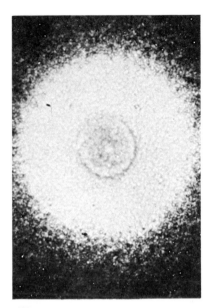

479

480

481 Mycoplasma colony. The colonial morphology is distinctive and may be used for preliminary identification. On cross-section the colony has the outline of a drawing pin. The central portion is dense, partly because of the growth of organisms in the interstices of the agar gel and partly because of heaping of organisms on the surface. The peripheral zone is thin and confined to the surface of the agar.

Diseases associated with *Mycoplasma pneumoniae*

Acute respiratory disease

Mycoplasma pneumoniae may cause outbreaks of acute respiratory disease, particularly in enclosed communities. Epidemics may occur at irregular intervals among the general population. Stevens–Johnson syndrome may be associated with mycoplasmal infection. Myringitis bullosa is a rare manifestation in which haemorrhagic bullae are found on the ear drum.

During the course of the illness antibodies against the mycoplasma develop and can be demonstrated by complement fixation, neutralisation, or immune fluorescence. In addition, many patients produce agglutinins that react with *Streptococcus MG* and with human group O erythrocytes at low temperatures.

482 Histology of lung in mycoplasmal pneumonia (haematoxylin and eosin stain). During the acute stage there is widespread inflammation of the lung parenchyma, and the alveolar walls are thickened with infiltrate. Bronchitis and bronchiolitis are prominent features, and there may be ulceration of the mucosa. Plugs of mucopus and debris may block the lumina of bronchioles, causing collapse of some alveoli and compensatory distension of others. The inflammatory exudate consists mainly of mononuclear and red blood cells. The section opposite shows a characteristic appearance in the late stage of the disease, with numerous lymphoid follicles adjacent to a bronchiole. (A = bronchus, B = lymphoid follicle, C = alveolus.)

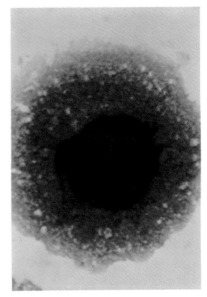

481

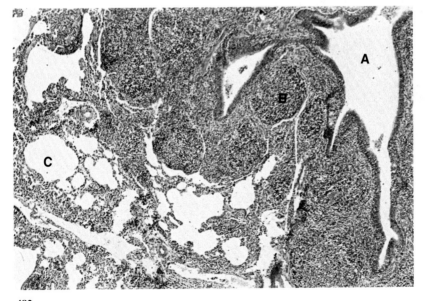

482

395

483 Radiograph of chest – peribronchial congestion. Onset of illness is gradual with general symptoms of headache, shivering, myalgia, and notable lassitude. Within a day or two the patient develops signs of an upper respiratory infection with an inflamed throat, followed by a distressing cough and retrosternal discomfort from tracheobronchitis. The sputum is scanty and may be mucoid or mucopurulent. Occasionally there may be streaks of blood. Radiography of the chest in such patients may show streaky shadowing from peribronchial congestion.

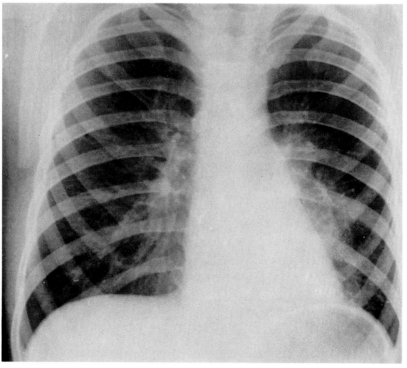

483

484 Radiograph of chest – lobular infection. The severity of the illness and the extent of pulmonary infection vary greatly. The main features are fever, malaise and undue tiredness. Respiratory distress is unusual and little can be found on clinical examination of the chest, apart from a few crepitations. Blockage of bronchioles, resulting in small areas of atelectasis, and spread of inflammation into the lung tissue around the bronchioles, are manifest as soft miliary shadowing or fine nodular mottling on chest radiographs.

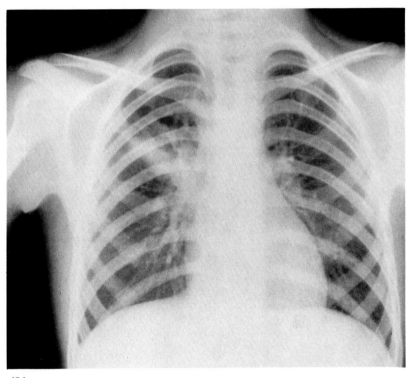

484

485 Radiograph of chest – hilar flare. In some cases radiography will show opacities with a ground-glass appearance fanning out from the hilum. This finding is not confined to mycoplasmal infection but can be caused by the psittacosis/ornithosis agent, *Coxiella burnetti*, and a number of viruses, including respiratory syncytial virus, adenovirus, parainfluenza virus, and influenza virus. For a definitive diagnosis it is necessary to demonstrate a fourfold rise in antibody against the suspected agent. Complement-fixation tests are commonly used; although not as sensitive as other antibody tests in mycoplasmal infections, they have the advantage of simplicity. Up to 50% of patients with mycoplasma pneumonia develop cold agglutinins against human type O red blood cells and over 60% may also possess agglutinating antibody against *Streptococcus MG*.

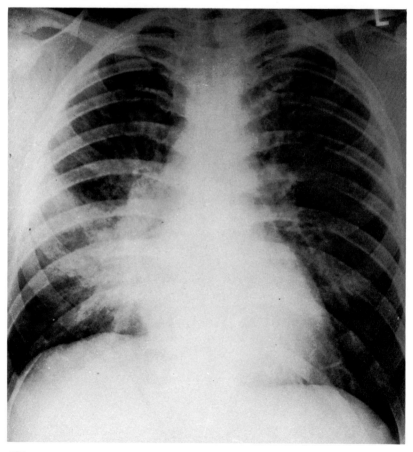

485

486 Radiograph of chest – lobar infection. The appearance of the lungs on radiographic examination varies considerably and does not match the clinical state. The shadows may be discrete and scattered throughout both lungs, or may be confluent and confined to one lobe, especially the lower. Occasionally the shadows migrate from one area to another.

The white blood cell count is usually normal but may be increased to 15×10^9/l. In at least 40% of cases the erythrocyte sedimentation rate exceeds 80 mm/hour. Although the illness follows a benign course, recovery is slow and radiological changes may persist for weeks. Death is rare; complications (which are uncommon) include haemolytic anaemia, encephalitis, myelitis, polyneuritis, myocarditis and arthritis.

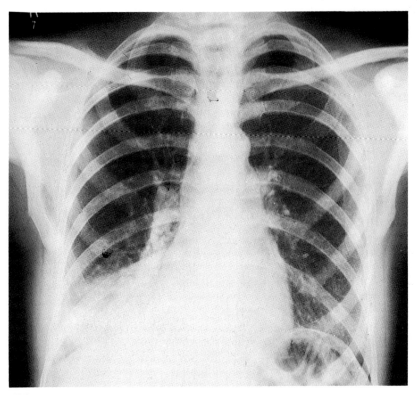

486

Stevens–Johnson syndrome

487 Mycoplasma and Stevens–Johnson syndrome. *Mycoplasma pneumoniae* may give rise to Stevens–Johnson syndrome with or without evidence of pulmonary infection. The fully developed syndrome consists of conjunctivitis, stomatitis, vulvitis or urethritis, and a pleomorphic rash (see **489–492**).

The conjunctivae are acutely inflamed, and the eyelids may be stuck together with congealed pus. When the mouth is severely affected there may be extensive ulceration and swallowing is painful. Towards the end of the second week the mucocutaneous lesions begin to heal, and the patient's general condition improves rapidly.

488 Mycoplasma and Stevens–Johnson syndrome. *Mycoplasma pneumoniae* has been recovered from patients with Stevens–Johnson syndrome. Because the dermis and epidermis are both affected there is considerable variation in the clinical appearance of the lesions. There is notable oedema of the dermis and heavy infiltration with neutrophil and eosinophil leucocytes. The small blood vessels are dilated and surrounded by lymphocytes. Vesicles may form both in the epidermis and in the dermis. Subepidermal vesicles may coalesce to form large bullae. The centre of the lesions may be discoloured by haemorrhage.

The typical target appearance is seen on the two skin lesions in this illustration. A large bulla rests on an erythematous base, and a dark area of haemorrhage is present in the centre.

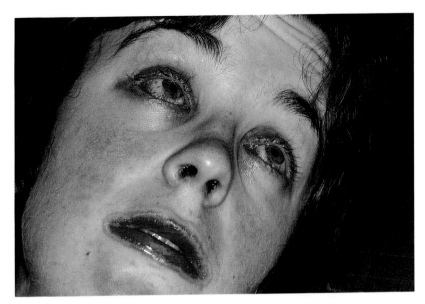

487

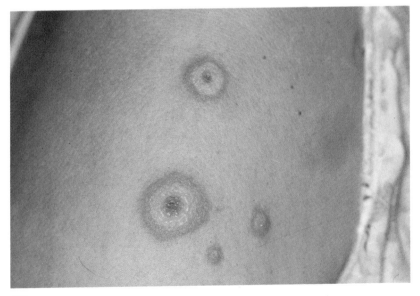

488

Stevens–Johnson syndrome

The Stevens–Johnson syndrome consists of a combination of a pleomorphic rash with ulceration of the mouth and inflammatory lesions of the eye and urethra. it is a condition of acute hypersensitivity and probably a severe variant of erythema multiforme. The precipitating factor may be an infection, particularly of the throat, or the syndrome may follow the use of drugs, such as sulphonamides or antibiotics (see also **487** and **488**).

489   Stevens–Johnson syndrome – mouth and buccal cavity. The illness usually begins with fever and some general malaise, followed by lesions on mucous membranes and skin. The stomatitis is particularly distressing because the mouth ulcers are painful and tend to bleed. The lips are often black with congealed blood and there may be difficulty in opening the mouth. When the buccal cavity and pharynx are severely ulcerated swallowing becomes an ordeal. Ulceration may extend into the trachea and bronchi and may be accompanied by pneumonia.

490   Stevens–Johnson syndrome – eyes. There is intense inflammation of the conjunctiva and the eyelids are often stuck together with pus.

Urethritis causes pain on micturition and lesions are usually present on the external genitalia. The patient remains acutely ill for a week or 10 days before the disease gradually resolves.

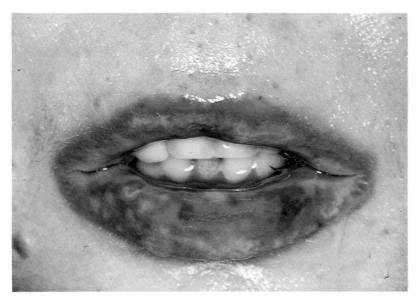

489

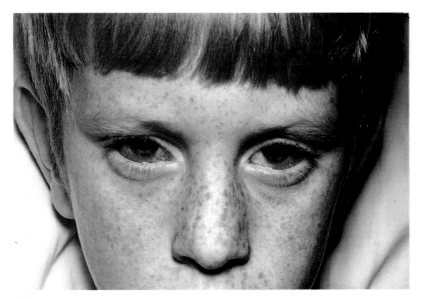

490

491 Stevens–Johnson syndrome – rash on trunk. The rash may precede or follow the other features. In mild cases the eruption appears on the extensor surfaces of the limbs and on the dorsum of the hands and feet; in more severe cases it involves the trunk, neck and head, and even the palms and soles. The scalp is rarely affected. Centrifugal distribution of the rash may closely resemble that of smallpox and used to cause difficulty in differential diagnosis. Some rashes are morbilliform but they do not evolve from above downwards; extensor surfaces are much more heavily affected than in measles (see **386** and **393**).

492 Stevens–Johnson syndrome – close up of rash. The typical eruption consists of circular erythematous lesions with concentric rings of different colours. These target or iris lesions measure about 1 cm in diameter and appear chiefly on the extremities. The rash is very variable and may consist of erythematous patches, vesicles, pustules and bullae in different combinations. Blood may escape into some of the lesions, altering the colour.

On histological examination of the skin the small blood vessels are congested and surrounded by mononuclear cells. Fluid exudate disrupts the cell layers, producing papules, vesicles and bullae.

493 Stevens–Johnson syndrome – arthritis. Many other structures may be affected in addition to the skin and mucous membranes. Pneumonia is a common complication, and myocarditis, pericarditis, encephalitis, and enteritis occur occasionally. This patient with Stevens–Johnson syndrome had painful swelling of the small joints of her hands during the acute stage of the rash. The arthritis persisted for a few weeks and then subsided, leaving no residual disability.

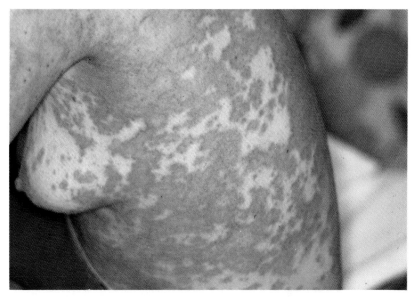

491

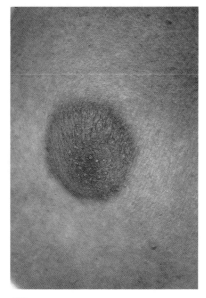

492

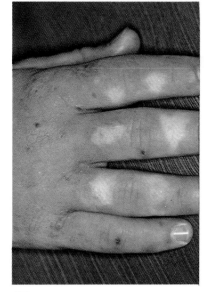

493

Scalded-skin syndrome (toxic epidermal necrolysis)

Scalded-skin syndrome (toxic epidermal necrolysis) resembles Stevens–Johnson syndrome but differs in respect of skin lesions. These are extremely painful and consist of large patches of necrotic epidermis, which slide off the underlying skin at the slightest pressure, leaving extensive raw areas. The overall picture is that of scalding.

There appear to be two types of scalded-skin syndrome: one induced by drugs and the other by infection with *Staphylococcus aureus*, usually of phage group II. The cleavage in necrolysis induced by drugs takes place in the subepidermal layers, whereas in staphylococcal infection it occurs within the epidermis. The staphylococcal form affects younger age groups and has a lower mortality rate. The strains of staphylococci associated with scalded-skin syndrome are those causing impetigo, pemphigus neonatorum, and Ritter's disease (see **47** and **48**). The staphylococcus may be present on the skin or other sites and produces an exotoxin (exfoliatin), which is responsible for the necrolysis.

494 Scalded-skin syndrome – lesions on face. This skin has a scalded appearance. The surface layer of the epidermis has separated and slid over the deeper layer, producing a wrinkled effect. The lips are acutely inflamed and crusted.

495 Scalded-skin syndrome – destructive effects. Necrolysis in the subepidermal layers may result in permanent damage to the skin. This child had a severe attack during which her right eyebrow slid on to her forehead before separating with the necrotic skin. The patient survived the acute stage, but the hairs of the eyebrows did not regenerate and keloid scars developed elsewhere.

496 Scalded-skin syndrome – Indian woman. The intense conjunctival congestion may be accompanied by keratitis, which may leave scarring and impaired vision. The surface epidermis has sheared off the skin on the eyelids; the lips are ulcerated and covered with dark scabs, where they have bled. The buccal cavity was extensively ulcerated.

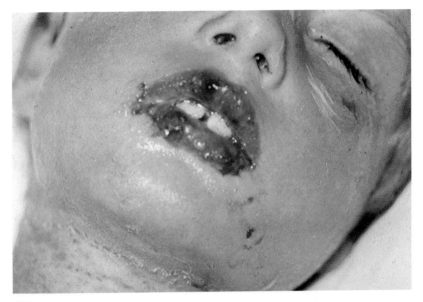

494

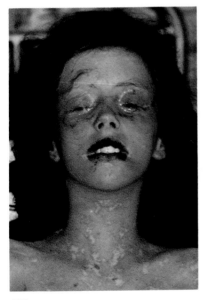

495

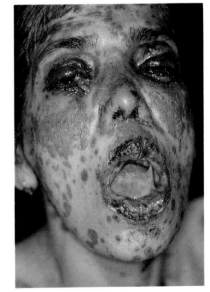

496

497 Scalded-skin syndrome – lesions on trunk. The surface pigmented layers may be shed during the acute stage in dark-skinned patients, but the colour of the skin is restored to normal during convalescence.

498 Scalded-skin syndrome – close-up of skin. The necrotic epidermis slides off the underlying skin at the slightest pressure. This constitutes Nikolsky's sign, which is not pathognomonic but may be found in other skin diseases such as pemphigus.

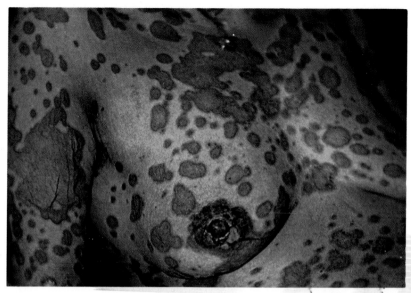

497

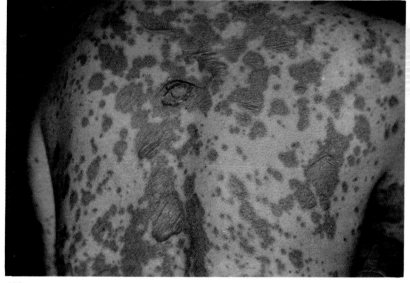

498

409

Pityriasis rosea

Pityriasis rosea is thought to be caused by a viral infection, but the agent has not yet been identified. Older children and young adults are predominantly affected. The main eruption is commonly preceded by a herald patch, that may appear 7–10 days before the rash emerges elsewhere. In the early stages of the illness there may be slight reddening of the throat and minimal enlargement of the cervical lymph nodes, but general disturbance is trivial. The rash disappears within 4–8 weeks from onset.

499 Pityriasis rosea – herald patch and general rash. The herald patch consists of a solitary scaly red macule, which usually appears on the trunk but is sometimes found on the neck or proximal parts of the limbs. It enlarges rapidly and may eventually measure 3–4 cm in length. There may be temporary loss of pigmentation on dark skins.

The rash elsewhere consists of scaly oval macules and rounded follicular papules. Over the thorax the long axes of the oval macules tend to follow the lines of the ribs. Lesions are scanty on the periphery of the limbs. The roseolar rash of secondary syphilis may simulate pityriasis rosea, but the presence of a herald patch and the absence of mucosal lesions should indicate the correct diagnosis.

500 Pityriasis rosea – components of rash. The rash is composed of two types of lesion: small red papules and characteristic pink oval macules, measuring 1–2 cm in length. After a few days the macules begin to desquamate from the centre outwards and form a collarette of scales with the free edges towards the centre. The rash is variable and the papular elements sometimes dominate; there may be slight itching.

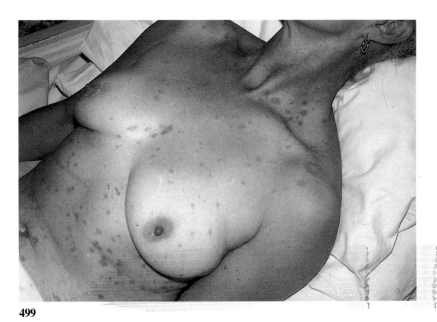

499

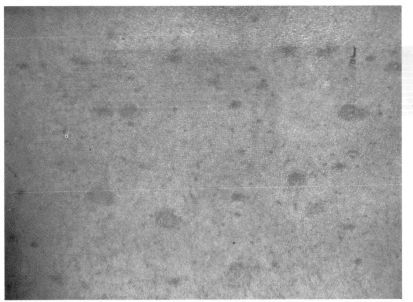

500

Kawasaki disease

Kawasaki disease, also called mucocutaneous lymph node syndrome, affects children and has been reported from many countries, but particularly Japan, where it was first described. The aetiology is unknown, though the disease is believed to be caused by an infectious agent. There are no specific tests and the diagnosis is established clinically when five out of the folloing six criterial have been met:

1 Fever of unknown aetiology
   - Lasting 5 days or longer
   - Unresponsive to antibiotics
2 Conjunctivae – bilateral congestion
3 Lips and mouth
   - Lips dry with redness and fissuring
   - Tongue – 'strawberry' appearance
   - Oropharynx – diffuse redness of the mucosa
4 Periphery of limbs
   - Early stage – redness of palms and soles with accompanying oedema of the dorsum of the hands and feet
   - Late stage – membranous desquamation beginning around the finger tips
5 Exanthem – pleomorphic rash most prominent on the trunk, absence of vesicles and crusts
6 Lymphadenopathy – acute non-suppurative enlargement of cervical nodes

501   Kawasaki disease – conjunctiva. Bilateral conjunctivitis is present in about 90% of cases. The bulbar conjunctivae are most severely affected but the palpebral conjunctivae may also be slightly congested.

502   Kawasaki disease – lips. The same proportion (90%) of patients have dry, reddened, cracked lips.

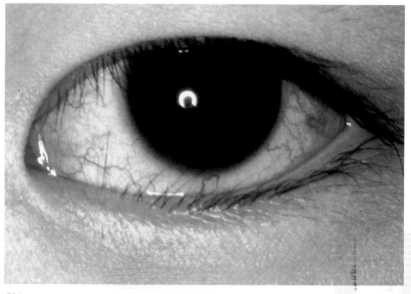

501

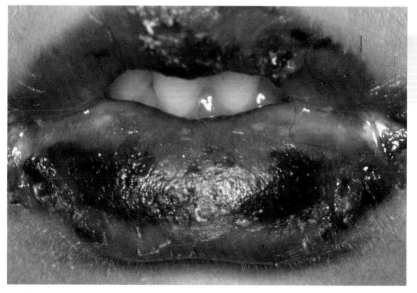

502

413

503 Kawasaki disease – tongue. The mucous membrane of the mouth and throat is reddened and dry, and the tongue with prominent red papillae closely resembles the peeled strawberry tongue of scarlet fever.

504 Kawasaki disease – lymph nodes. The cervical lymph nodes are enlarged, firm, and slightly tender. They do not suppurate.

505 Kawasaki disease – exanthem. A rash appears within a few days of onset of scarlet fever and usually persists for about a week. It is most prominent over the trunk, but may extend to the face and limbs. It is erythematous and may simulate the exanthem of measles or erythema multiforme.

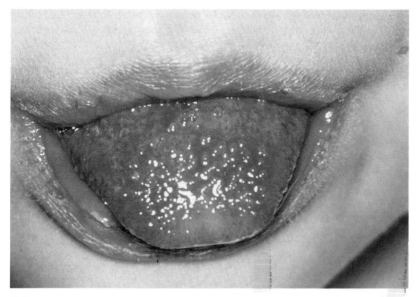

503

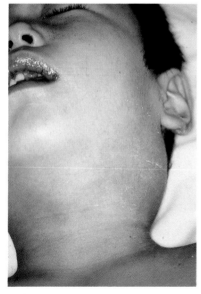

504

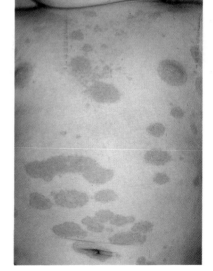

505

506 Kawasaki disease – extremities. Indurative oedema of the dorsum of the hands and feet is an early feature and may be accompanied by flushing of the palms and soles.

507 Kawasaki disease – membranous desquamation. During the second or third week of illness the skin begins to peel around the nail folds, and large strips of skin may separate from the fingers.

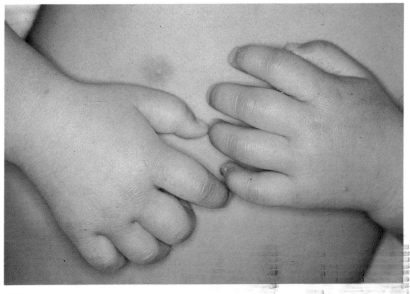

506

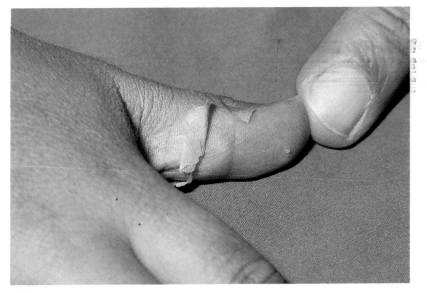

507

417

508 Kawasaki disease – coronary artery thrombosis. Carditis is a common finding and the main cause of death. It may be associated with angiitis of the coronary vessels resulting in aneurysm and thrombosis. The prognosis is worst in boys under 1 year of age, who have prolonged fever and a rash accompanied by a very high erythrocyte sedimentation rate. Pronounced thrombocytosis is common during the second and third weeks of illness and may predispose the patient to thrombosis. Mortality is between 1 and 2%.

509 Kawasaki disease – coronary angiography. Abnormal coronary arteries were shown in about 60% of the patients studied in one series. Some patients were found to have aneurysms; others were found to have irregular, tortuous, or stenosed arteries. The angiographic appearances returned to normal in a few patients.

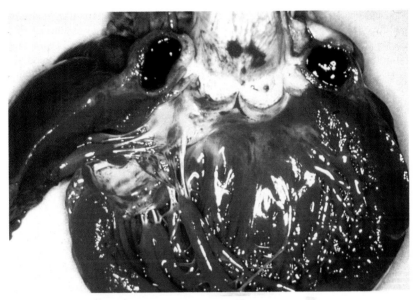

508

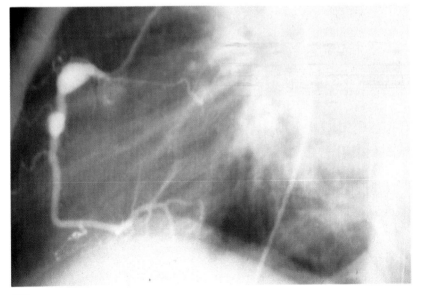

509

510 Kawasaki disease – hydrops of gallbladder. Diarrhoea and abdominal pain may occur at any stage of the illness. In some patients the abdominal discomfort may be associated with hydrops of the gallbladder, which has been demonstrated here by ultrasonography. In this child the hydrops resolved spontaneously. Other features found occasionally include meningitis, arthritis, urethritis, and otitis media. (A = liver, B = gallbladder, C = kidney.)

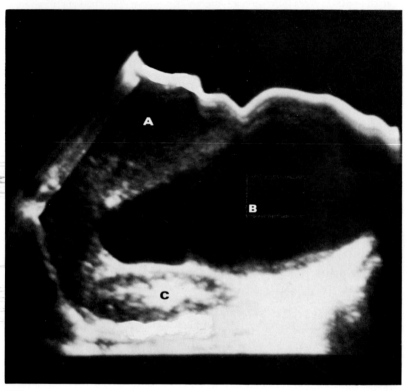

510

Cat-scratch disease

Cat-scratch disease is generally acquired as a result of a scratch, lick or bite from an apparently healthy cat. Within a few days a primary lesion develops at the site of injury. This local reaction usually takes the form of a reddened papule, but may be vesicular or crusted. Occasionally there is no local response. After an interval of 10–30 days the regional lymph nodes become enlarged and there may be slight constitutional disturbance with malaise and low-grade fever. The subsequent course of the illness is variable and may be prolonged. Occasionally the illness may follow a more severe course with encephalitis, follicular conjunctivitis or retinitis. When the illness is uncomplicated ultimate recovery is assured and death is unknown.

Two bacteria have so far been cultured independently from patients with cat-scratch disease – *Afipia felis*, a motile Gram-negative bacillus, and the unrelated *Rochalimaea henselae*, a member of the alpha-2 subgroup of the class Proteabacteria. The latter is more commonly associated with the disease.

511 Histology of lymph node (haematoxylin and eosin stain). Initially there is hypoplasia of the reticulum, but necrotic foci soon appear in the germinal follicles and break down to form micro-abscesses, which coalesce and may discharge on the surface of the skin. The foci of necrotic material are surrounded by a layer of epithelioid cells interspersed by giant cells of Langhans type. The necrotic areas in the lymph node section shown here have stained a bright pink.

512 Enlarged supraclavicular and infraclavicular lymph nodes. When suppuration is absent the swelling may subside in 2 or 3 weeks; when it is gross, regression may take 2 or 3 months. The nature of the infection may be overlooked when the primary component is missing, but the possibility of cat-scratch disease should always be considered when there is a history of exposure to cats in a patient with unexplained persistent lymphadenitis. A clinical diagnosis may not be possible with an atypical presentation, such as encephalitis. Confirmation of the diagnosis rests with the specific skin test using an antigen prepared from sterilised dilute pus from a bubo, culture of lymph node material for *A. felis* or *R. henselae*, and antibody tests, when available, on paired sera.

513 Enlarged epitrochlear and infraclavicular lymph nodes. The epitrochlear, axillary and cervical groups are most commonly affected. The swollen nodes are mobile and vary in consistency with the degree of suppuration; some are tender. The overlying skin is usually normal but may be inflamed and sometimes breaks down to form a discharging sinus. Lymphangitis is not a feature.

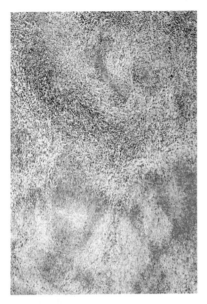

511

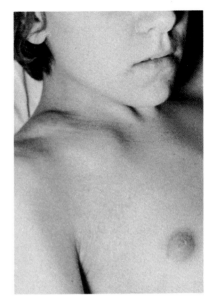

512

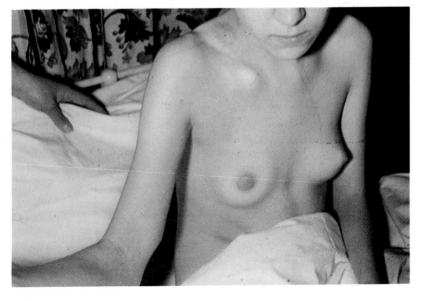

513

INDEX

*(The references printed in **bold** type are to picture and caption numbers, those in light type are to page numbers.)*